ONCOLOGY

International Journal of Cancer Research and Treatment

Founded 1948 as 'Oncologia' by H.R. Schinz
Continued by V. Richards 1967–1975

KARGER

Printed in Switzerland
on acid-free paper by
Druckerei Schüler AG, Biel

Appears bimonthly:
1 volume per year (6 issues)

ONCOLOGY

Submission: Only original papers written in English are considered and should be sent to:

S. Karger AG
Editorial Dept. 'Oncology'
P.O. Box
CH-4009 Basel (Switzerland)

Manuscripts should be submitted in triplicate (with three sets of illustrations of which one is an original), typewritten double-spaced on one side of the paper, with a wide margin.

Conditions: All manuscripts are subject to editorial review. The editors reserve the right to improve style and, if necessary, return the manuscript for re-writing to the author. Submission of an article for publication implies the transfer of the copyright from the author to the publisher upon acceptance. Accepted papers become the permanent property of 'Oncology' and may not be reproduced by any means, in whole or in part, without the written consent of the publisher. It is the author's responsibility to obtain permission to reproduce illustrations, tables, etc. from other publications.

Arrangement

Title page: The first page of each paper should indicate the title (main title underlined), the authors' names, and the institute where the work was conducted. A short title for use as running head as well as the full address of the author to whom correspondence should be sent are also required.

Full address: The exact postal address complete with postal code must be given at the bottom of the title page. Please also supply Phone and Fax numbers.

Key words: For indexing purposes, a list of 3-10 key words in English is essential.

Abstract: Each paper needs an abstract of up to 10 lines.

Small type: Paragraphs which can or must be set in smaller type (case histories, test methods, etc.) should be indicated with a 'p' (petit) in the margin on the left-hand side.

Footnotes: Avoid footnotes. When essential, they are numbered consecutively and typed at the foot of the appropriate page.

Tables and illustrations: Tables and illustrations (both numbered in Arabic numerals) should be prepared on separate sheets. Tables require a heading and figures a legend, also prepared on a separate sheet. For the reproduction of illustrations, only good drawings and original photographs can be accepted; negatives or photocopies cannot be used. When possible, group several illustrations on one block for reproduction (max. size 181 × 223 mm) or provide crop marks. On the back of each illustration, indicate its number, the author's name, and 'top'. Color illustrations are reproduced at the author's expense.

References: In the text identify references by Arabic numerals [in square brackets]. Material submitted for publication but not yet accepted should be noted as 'unpublished data' and not be included in the reference list. The list of references should include only those publications which are cited in the text. Do not alphabetize; number references in the order in which they are first mentioned in the text. The surnames of the authors followed by initials should be given. There should be no punctuation other than a comma to separate the authors. Cite all authors, 'et al' is not sufficient. Abbreviate journal names according to the Index Medicus system. (Also see International Committee of Medical Journal Editors: Uniform requirements for manuscripts submitted to biomedical journals. Br Med J 1988;296:401-405.)

Examples

(a) Papers published in periodicals: Kauffman HF, van der Heide S, Beaumont F, Blok H, de Vries K: Class-specific antibody determination against *Aspergillus fumigatus* by means of the enzyme-linked immunosorbent assay. III. Comparative study: IgG, IgA, IgM ELISA titers, precipitating antibodies and IgE binding after fractionation of the antigen. Int Arch Allergy Appl Immunol 1986;80:300-306.

(b) Monographs: Matthews DE, Farewell VT: Using and Understanding Medical Statistics. Basel, Karger, 1985.

(c) Edited books: Hardy WD Jr, Essex M: FeLV-induced feline acquired immune deficiency syndrome: A model for human AIDS; in Klein E (ed): Acquired Immunodeficiency Syndrome. Prog Allergy. Basel, Karger, 1986, vol 37, pp 353-376.

Further details: Authors may consult our leaflet 'Rules for the Preparation of Manuscripts', available on request from the Publisher, S. Karger AG, P.O. Box, CH-4009 Basel (Switzerland).

Page charges: There is no page charge for papers of 3 or fewer printed pages (including tables, illustrations and references). Each additional complete or partial page is charged to the author at SFr. 225.– / US$ 150.00. The allotted size of a paper is equal to approx. 9 manuscript pages (including tables, illustrations and references).

Galley proofs: Unless indicated otherwise, galley proofs are sent to the first-named author and should be returned with the least possible delay. Alterations made in galley proofs, other than the correction of printer's errors, are charged to the author. No page proofs are supplied.

Reprints: Order forms and a price list are sent with the galley proofs. Orders submitted after the issue is printed are subject to considerably higher prices. Allow five weeks from date of publication for delivery of reprints.

KARGER

General Information — ONCOLOGY

Publication data: 'Oncology' is published 6 times annually. Volume 50 with 6 issues appears in 1993.

Subscription rates: Subscriptions run for a full calendar year. Prices are given per volume.

Personal subscription:

Subscription + postage and handling

SFr. 555.10 + SFr. 16.80 Europe

SFr. 555.10 + SFr. 25.20 Overseas

US$ 370.30 + US$ 16.80

(Must be in the name of, billed to, and paid by an individual. Order must be marked 'personal subscription'.)

Institutional subscription:

Subscription + postage and handling

SFr. 793.– + SFr. 24.– Europe

SFr. 793.– + SFr. 36.– Overseas

US$ 529.00 + US$ 24.00

Airmail postage: SFr. 36.–, US$ 30.00. (Extra per volume.)

Microform edition: SFr. 396.50, US$ 264.50. (Available exclusively to subscribers of the paper edition.)

Advertising: Correspondence and rate requests should be addressed to the Publisher.

Subscription orders: Orders can be placed at agencies, bookstores, directly with the Publisher S. Karger AG, P.O. Box, CH–4009 Basel (Switzerland) or with any of the following distributors:

Deutschland: S. Karger GmbH
Lörracher Strasse 16A, Postfach
D-W-7800 Freiburg

France: Librairie Luginbühl
36, bd de Latour-Maubourg, F-75007 Paris

Great Britain, Ireland: S. Karger Publishers
11 Ravenscroft Road
Beckenham, Kent BR3 4TP

USA: S. Karger Publishers, Inc.
26 West Avon Road, P.O. Box 529
Farmington, CT 06085

India, Bangladesh, Sri Lanka:
S. Karger India Subscription Agency
B-5/132 Safdarjung Enclave
New Delhi-110029

Japan: Katakura Libri, Inc.
36-9 Hongo 3-chome, Bunkyo-ku, Tokyo 113

Change of address: Both old and new address should be sent to the subscription source.

Single issues and back volumes: Information can be obtained through the Publisher.

Bibliographic indices: This journal is regularly listed in bibliographic services, including *Current Contents®*.

Book Reviews: Books are accepted for review by special agreement.

KARGER

Contributions to Oncology/Beiträge zur Onkologie
(ISSN 0250–3220), **Vol. 44**
Series Editors: H. Huber, Innsbruck; W. Queisser, Mannheim

Metastasis: Basic Research and Its Clinical Applications

Editors:
H. Rabes
P.E. Peters
K. Munk

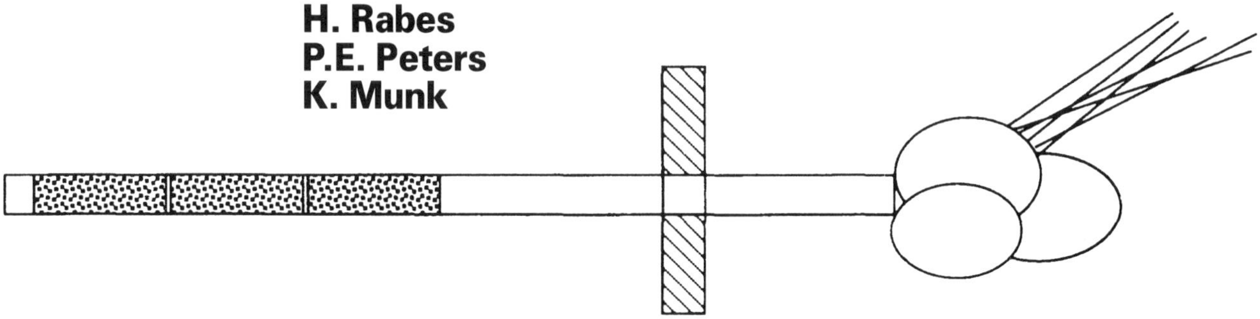

An interdisciplinary perspective

Metastasis is still the leading cause of death in cancer patients. In order to improve the prevention and treatment of metastasis, the basic principles and mechanisms of this complex process need to be elucidated. This volume contains the reports of internationally renowned scientists and clinicians on recent progress in metastasis research and its clinical applications. The contributions detail what is now known about the basic processes of metastasis and the specific cellular components, extracellular factors and genes that are involved. The implications of this new knowledge for impeding steps in the metastatic cascade are also discussed.
Bringing together findings from theoretical, experimental and clinical metastasis research, this book provides readers with a thorough overview of current efforts to meet the many challenges posed by metastasis.

Main Headings

Concepts, Genetic Aspects and Models
Molecular Mechanisms and Modulation of Invasion and Metastasis
Growth Factors, Angiogenesis, Microvasculature and Metastasis
Aspects of Metastatic Melanoma
Immunological Aspects and Therapeutic Approaches
New Methods in Radiological Diagnosis, Therapy Planning and Therapy of Metastasis

Fields of Interest

Oncology; Cell Biology, Genetics, Immunology, Molecular Biology, Pathology, Radiology

Contributions to Oncology/Beiträge zur Onkologie, Vol. 44
Metastasis: Basic Research and Its Clinical Applications
8th International Expert Meeting of the Dr. Mildred Scheel-Stiftung für Krebsforschung, Bonn, October 1991
Editors: Rabes, H. (München); Peters, P.E. (Münster); Munk, K. (Heidelberg)
X + 394 p., 65 fig., 43 tab., hard cover, 1992
SFr. 79.– / DM 95.– / £ 39.50 / US $ 63.25
Prices subject to change
DM price for FRG, £ price for UK, US $ price for USA only
ISBN 3–8055–5610–1

Ondansetron – Global Experience and Future Potential

Ondansetron – Global Experience and Future Potential

Satellite Symposium held during the 17th Congress of the European Society for Medical Oncology
November 7–10, 1992
Lyon, France

Guest Editors
M. Soukop, Glasgow
K. Cunningham, London

27 figures and 15 tables, 1993

KARGER

S. Karger
Medical and Scientific Publishers
Basel · Freiburg · Paris · London
New York · New Delhi · Bangkok
Singapore · Tokyo · Sydney

Drug Dosage
The authors and the publisher have exerted every effort to ensure that drug selection and dosage set forth in this text are in accord with current recommendations and practice at the time of publication. However, in view of ongoing research, changes in government regulations, and the constant flow of information relating to drug therapy and drug reactions, the reader is urged to check the package insert for each drug for any change in indications and dosage and for added warnings and precautions. This is particularly important when the recommended agent is a new and/or infrequently employed drug.

P.O. Box, CH-4009 Basel (Switzerland)
Printed in Switzerland on acid-free paper by
Graphische Anstalt Schüler AG, Biel
ISBN 3-8055-5783-3

Contents

M. Marty

Introduction

Ondansetron, the first highly selective 5-HT_3 receptor antagonist to reach the market, is now approved (as ondansetron hydrochloride dihydrate) for use in over 70 countries worldwide. After 3 years of clinical use and over 4 million patient treatments ondansetron has established an important role in cancer therapy and represents a real advance in the management of chemotherapy- and radiotherapy-induced emesis. Since the submission of the clinical dossier to regulatory authorities in April 1989, clinical experience with ondansetron has grown considerably. For example, it is now well established that a single intravenous dose of ondansetron is as effective as the dose regimens used in the initial clinical studies [1] and that twice daily oral dosing is as effective as a 3-times-a-day schedule [2]. It is therefore timely to review more recent clinical trial data and the global experience with ondansetron to help us to use this agent in an optimal manner and to look ahead to the future potential of ondansetron in cancer therapy.

References

1 Brown GW, Paes D, Bryson J, Freeman AJ: The effectiveness of a single intravenous dose of ondansetron. Oncology 1992;49:273–278.

2 Dicato MA, Kaasa S, Campora E, Bleiberg H, Warnier P, Vindovoghel A, Cunningham D, Liebhard A, Upadhyaya BK: Efficacy of twice daily versus three times daily oral ondansetron in the prevention of chemotherapy induced emesis: A randomised, single blind, multicentre study. Clin Oncol 1992;4:275–279.

Oncology 1993;50:159–162

M. Marty

Department of Medical Oncology,
Hospital Saint Louis, Paris, France

Future Trends in Cancer Treatment and Emesis Control

Key Words
Ondansetron
Chemotherapy
Chemoprotective agents
Dose intensification

Abstract
The treatment of cancer patients has improved over the last few years for a variety of reasons. These include improvements in diagnosis, more potent chemotherapeutic drugs and the introduction of new ways of containing or eliminating cancers by the use of multi-modality treatment regimens often facilitated by the use of chemoprotective agents. Cancer patients have also benefited from an increased awareness of their needs, with health care professionals paying attention to toxicities of treatment and optimising treatment schedules to combine the best possible medical outcome with patient comfort and acceptability of treatment. Thus not all the advances seen in the management of cancer patients have relied upon the introduction of novel antitumour agents; important advances have been made by the optimal use of existing drugs, the revision of treatment schedules and better control of the side effects of treatment. One of the more distressing side effects of cancer chemotherapy, having a profound effect on its acceptability to patients, is nausea and vomiting. The introduction over the last 3 years, of ondansetron, the first generally available 5-HT_3 receptor antagonist, has had beneficial effects on the management of patients. Through improvements in anti-emetic control ondansetron has provided a better quality of life and is now beginning to impact on the design and administration of conventional chemotherapy treatment schedules. This paper reviews the changes that have been seen with the use of ondansetron and makes several suggestions about areas where clinicians might find a beneficial role for 5-HT_3 receptor antagonists.

Background

Chemotherapy has a prominent role in the whole armamentarium of available cancer treatments. Around 80–90% of cancer patients will expect to receive some form of chemotherapy – as primary treatment for their disease, as adjuvant therapy to local regional treatment or as a palliative measure as the disease progresses. Furthermore most patients will be exposed to several different chemotherapy regimens; anything from 1 to 4 different combinations may be given to an individual. Chemotherapy-induced emesis is widespread, its severity and duration vary with the nature of the chemotherapy. Cisplatin is universally acknowledged to be the most highly emetogenic agent and the majority of non-cisplatin chemotherapy regimens will contain cyclophosphamide, doxorubicin or dacarbazine which have been shown to induce nausea and vomiting in 60–80% of cases. It is important,

Prof. M. Marty
Department of Medical Oncology
Hospital Saint Louis
F–75010 Paris (France)

therefore, to consider the effects and implications of such chemotherapy-induced emesis. The main emesis-related problems encountered are: electrolyte imbalance, alterations in chemotherapy regimens and an effect of increasing hospital costs.

Electrolyte Imbalance

Constant loss of electrolytes in the vomitus can lead to electrolyte imbalance. This can usually be well monitored and controlled in hospitalised patients before it becomes a clinical problem but it may be more hazardous in outpatients, especially the elderly.

Alterations in Chemotherapy Regimens

Severe nausea and vomiting cause such distress that chemotherapy regimens may have to be adjusted. Lower doses of the emetogenic agent may be given or the agent(s) may be replaced by a drug or drugs with lower toxicity but less clinical efficacy. Sometimes expensive analogues of certain chemotherapy drugs will be used in an attempt to circumvent side effects.

Patients may delay outpatient appointments beyond the optimum timing for treatment and/or severe nausea and vomiting may result in withdrawal from active treatment altogether. Up to 20% of patients have been reported to withdraw from treatment through nausea and vomiting. Poor adherence to treatment schedules can adversely affect clinical outcome. In cases where palliation is all that can be offered to the patient, it is clearly especially important that patients do not withdraw and that unpleasant side effects are avoided.

Cost Increases

The need to control chemotherapy-induced emesis necessarily involves drug costs. But there are also costs incurred when anti-emetic control is poor in terms of nursing time, laundry of soiled linen and longer stays in hospital. Nausea and vomiting therefore not only distress the patient but can influence an oncologist's decision about timing and doses of chemotherapy. Indirectly, nausea and vomiting can reduce the effectiveness of chemotherapy and add to the financial burden of an oncology unit.

Impact of Effective Anti-Emetic Control

As nausea and vomiting can have such detrimental effects on patient care the impact of improved anti-emetic control should be significant. Since its introduction ondansetron has been demonstrated to control nausea and vomiting in more than 70% of patients, and 80% of those who are free of nausea and vomiting will be adequately controlled for up to 3 courses of chemotherapy [1]. Even with highly emetogenic chemotherapy, such as cisplatin, ondansetron controls acute nausea and vomiting in up to 75% of patients [2]. Furthermore the addition of dexamethasone improves upon this level of efficacy [3, 4].

Patient Withdrawals

Improved anti-emetic control has been shown to reduce the number of patient withdrawals compared with standard anti-emetic regimens [1, 5, 6]. Such reduced withdrawal rates imply better compliance with treatment schedules and less need to alter or reduce chemotherapy regimens. While closer adherence to treatment schedules is only anecdotal at this stage, it is certainly worth investigating. Better compliance with treatment may allow more aggressive scheduling of treatment sessions, shortening of the inter-dose interval and thereby maintaining more constant, and/or higher, tissue levels of the cytotoxic drug.

Increased Efficiency of Chemotherapy

It is also possible that improved anti-emetic control can increase the efficiency of chemotherapy drugs by allowing faster drug infusions and increasing maximal plasma concentrations (C_{max}). The cytotoxic action of a drug when tested ex vivo is often linearly related to its concentration. Selection of a suitable clinical dose, however, involves other considerations and will frequently be limited by the side effects of the drug. Where nausea and vomiting are the limiting toxicity the use of ondansetron could have important therapeutic implications.

Improved Cost-Effectiveness

Better control of nausea and vomiting means that patients stay in hospital for shorter periods and clinicians and nurses are more confident in arranging discharge, transportation and homecare if a patient can be given effective anti-emetic therapy. Homecare is also easier with the availability of oral anti-emetics; this both improves patient comfort and reduces costs. Chemotherapy can be given over shorter periods and in a more efficient manner reducing the medical and nursing time necessary. Nursing care can also be provided more efficiently where patients are not suffering from nausea and vomiting.

Although more effective use of cytotoxic drugs could conceivably produce an increased drug bill in practice this

Table 1. Summary of conventional and possible increased dose regimens (in mg/m²) for some common cytotoxic drugs

Agent	Conventional	Intensified	High-dose	Massive-dose
Cyclophosphamide	600–1,000	1,000–1,200	1,200–1,500	>4–6,000
Ifosfamide	2–4,500	4,500–8,000	>8,000	?
Melphalan	30–50	?	?	140–180
Thiotepa	10–30	30–50	?	400–700
Cisplatin	50–80	80–120	>200	?
Carboplatin	250–400	400–600	600–800	800–1,200
Doxorubicin	30–50	50–75	75–90	90–135
Mitronanzone	10–14	14–20	?	40–60
Etoposide	300–450	450–600	?	100–1,500
Vincristine	1.4	1.4–2	NA	NA
Vinblastine	4–6	6–10	NA	NA
Methotrexate	40–80	80–500	500–8,000	>8,000

has not been found. Cheaper versions of some reference cytotoxic drugs can be used whereas previously more expensive analogues were used to avoid drug-induced nausea and vomiting. In one unit the number of medical interventions increased by 17% (utilising the same number of personnel) while drug costs only increased by 10% [5].

While the unit cost of ondansetron is higher than that for many anti-emetic drugs the comparison is really only valid if similar efficacy is obtained. Evaluation of the cost of ondansetron per successful treatment shows that it is no more expensive than other efficacious anti-emetics [7]. In many situations ondansetron, compared with other agents, gives superior anti-emetic control making the comparison with other regimens less meaningful.

Dose Intensification

A variety of chemoprotective agents have been available for some time and some more sophisticated agents have been introduced over recent years. These include the colony-stimulating factors: G-CSF and GM-CSF, stem cell factor, interleukin-3, erythropoietin, folinic acid, mesna and anti-emetics. The use of these agents will reduce the acute toxicity of chemotherapy drugs, e.g. neutropenia, nausea and vomiting, and also oppose subacute or chronic side effects such as anaemia, haemorrhagic cystitis, neurotoxicity, nephrotoxicity and cardiotoxicity.

The effective control of the side effects of chemotherapy drugs has allowed oncologists to try and improve success rates by increasing drug doses, decreasing inter-dose interval or a combination of both. Some agents, such as the vinca alkaloids and cisplatin are probably being utilised at the upper limit of their possible doses, but for many others increased or intensified doses are under investigation. Table 1 summarises the intensified doses that are currently under consideration. This table also shows some higher dose schedules that have been considered: 'high-dose' and 'massive-dose', where drug doses are up to 20 times those used in the conventional setting. These are becoming more widely investigated and used.

Intensified dosing has already been used in combination chemotherapy. For example, in the widely used FEC regimen (fluorouracil, epirubicin, cyclophosphamide) the epirubicin dose has been increased from 40–50 to 75–100 mg/m² and the cyclophosphamide/cisplatin regimen used to treat ovarian cancer has been increased to 1,000 mg/m² cyclophosphamide and 100 mg/m² cisplatin.

We are already seeing encouraging results with the use of intensified dosing. For example, a study of advanced breast cancer patients showed that for patients with stage III disease a longer disease-free survival was obtained in those patients receiving a higher dose intensity [8].

While results of dose intensification may still be controversial it seems that we can demonstrate better results from increased dose intensity in the areas of non-Hodgkin's lymphoma, myelomas, breast carcinoma, ovarian carcinoma and small cell lung cancer. It is of course likely that such dose intensification will produce a concomitant increase in side effects. While studies have yet to investigate this aspect of dose intensification the availability of effective chemoprotective agents will add to the development of this area of cytotoxic therapy.

New Chemotherapeutic Agents

Experience with chemoprotective agents, including anti-emetics, will mean that the toxicities of new drugs will not restrict their entry into clinical use as has previously been the case.

Oral Chemotherapy

Oral chemotherapy has a role to play in non-Hodgkin's lymphoma, breast carcinoma, ovarian carcinoma and small cell lung cancer. Data are few on how to control emesis adequately in patients receiving long-term oral chemotherapy. In many countries the majority of patients who receive such regimens are elderly and/or being treated in non-specialist units. Such patients are particularly vulnerable to the effects of dehydration and poor nutrition which may be exacerbated by poor anti-emetic control. Ondansetron has been demonstrated to control emesis in outpatients receiving oral chemotherapy [9], but these studies need extending.

Conclusions

It is possible to see that the introduction of the 5-HT_3 receptor antagonist ondansetron has had an important effect on the treatment of nausea and vomiting. It has also helped define the area in which we are unable to achieve total control of emesis and which requires further investigation. Indirectly the increased tolerance of many cytotoxic drugs has allowed more efficient use and scheduling of chemotherapy treatment and should have an important role to play as novel agents are introduced and chemotherapy regimens are refined.

References

1 Soukop M, McQuade B, Hunter E, Stewart A, Kaye S, Cassidy J, Kerr D, Khanna S, Smyth J, Coleman R, Cunningham D, Powles T, Davidson N, Hutcheon A, Green J, Slater A, Rustin G, Carney D: Ondansetron compared with metoclopramide in the control of emesis and quality of life during repeated chemotherapy. Oncology 1992;49:295–304.

2 Marty M, Pouillart P, Scholl S, Droz JP, Azab M, Brion N, Pujade-Lauraine E, Paule B, Paes D, Bons J: Comparison of the 5-hydroxytryptamine 3 (serotonin) antagonist ondansetron (GR 38032F) with high-dose metoclopramide in the control of cisplatin-induced emesis. N Engl J Med 1990;322:816–821.

3 Smyth JF, Coleman RE, Nicolson M, Gallmeier WM, Leonard RCF, Cornbleet MA, Allan SG, Upadhyaya BK, Bruntsch U: Does dexamethasone enhance control of acute cisplatin induced emesis by ondansetron? Br Med J 1991;303:1423–1426.

4 Roila F, Tonato M, Cognetti F, Cortesi E, Favalli G, Marangolo M, Amadori D, Bella MA, Gramazio V, Donati D, Ballatori E, Del Favero A: Prevention of cisplatin-induced emesis: A double blind multicentre randomised crossover study comparing ondansetron and ondansetron plus dexamethasone. J Clin Oncol 1991; 9:675–678.

5 Marty M: Ondansetron and chemotherapy induced emesis (editorial). 3rd Int Congr on Neo-Adjuvant Chemotherapy. Berlin, Springer, 1991, pp 3–7.

6 Depierre A, Lebeau B, d'Allens H: A comparison of ondansetron with alizapride plus methylprednisolone in the control of cisplatin-induced emesis. Oncology 1992;49:305–311.

7 Cunningham D, Gore M, Davidson N, Miocevich M, Manchanda M, Wells N: The real costs of emesis – An economic analysis of ondansetron vs. metoclopramide in controlling emesis in patients receiving chemotherapy for cancer. Eur J Cancer 1993;29A:303–306.

8 Ang PT, Buzdar AU, Smith TL, Kau S, Hortobagyi GN: Analysis of dose intensity in doxorubicin-containing adjuvant chemotherapy in stage II and III breast carcinoma. J Clin Oncol 1989;7:1677–1684.

9 Dicato MA, Kaasa S, Campora E, Bleiberg H, Warnier P, Vindovoghel A, Cunningham D, Liebhard A, Upadhyaya BK: Efficacy of twice daily versus three times daily oral ondansetron in the prevention of chemotherapy induced emesis: A randomised, single blind, multicentre study. Clin Oncol 1992;4:275–279

Oncology 1993;50:163–167

F. Roila

Medical Oncology Division, Polyclinic Hospital, Perugia, Italy

Ondansetron plus Dexamethasone Compared to the 'Standard' Metoclopramide Combination

Key Words
Cisplatin-induced emesis
Ondansetron
Dexamethasone
Metoclopramide
Diphenhydramine

Abstract

This paper describes a multicentre, double-blind, parallel group study which compared ondansetron (0.15 mg/kg i.v. × 3) plus dexamethasone (20 mg i.v.) with metoclopramide (3 mg/kg i.v. × 2) plus dexamethasone (20 mg i.v.) and diphenhydramine (50 mg i.v.) for the prevention of cisplatin-induced emesis and nausea. Two hundred and eighty-nine consecutive patients receiving chemotherapy containing cisplatin at doses ≥ 50 mg/m^2 entered the study and 267 patients were evaluable for efficacy. The ondansetron regimen was significantly superior compared with the metoclopramide regimen in the control of acute emesis and nausea. Ondansetron plus dexamethasone provided complete protection against retching and vomiting in 79% of patients compared with 59% of patients given the metoclopramide combination ($p < 0.002$). Similarly ondansetron plus dexamethasone completely prevented nausea in 77% of patients, whereas the metoclopramide combination protected 66% of patients ($p < 0.051$). Success (no nausea and no emesis) was afforded to 69% of those patients given ondansetron plus dexamethasone as opposed to 50% of patients given the metoclopramide combination ($p < 0.003$). From day 2–4 all patients received the same anti-emetic regimen of oral metoclopramide and intramuscular dexamethasone. Significantly fewer patients who had received the ondansetron regimen on day 1 vomited on days 2 and 3 compared with those who had received the triple drug combination (84–86 and 68–71%, respectively, $p < 0.006$). Nausea was also better controlled in this group on day 2. On subsequent cisplatin cycles, the incidence of acute vomiting rose to 53% in those patients given the metoclopramide regimen, but remained low (26%) in the group treated with ondansetron plus dexamethasone. Patients receiving the metoclopramide regimen had significantly more sedation than patients receiving ondansetron plus dexamethasone (12 vs. 2%; $p < 0.005$). Extrapyramidal reactions were only observed in metoclopramide-treated patients (3%). The results of this study suggest that ondansetron plus dexamethasone is a more effective and better tolerated anti-emetic regimen compared with metoclopramide plus dexamethasone and diphenhydramine for the prevention of acute cisplatin-induced emesis.

Presented on behalf of the Italian Group for Antiemetic Research (see Appendix for authors and participating centres).

F. Roila
Divisione Oncologia Medica
Ospedale Policlinico
I–06122 Perugia (Italy)

Table 1. Anti-emetic dose schedules day 1

Treatment	Before chemotherapy	After chemotherapy
A	ondansetron 0.15 mg/kg i.v. dexamethasone 20 mg i.v.	ondansetron 0.15 mg/kg i.v. 2 hourly × 2
B	metoclopramide 3 mg/kg i.v. dexamethasone 20 mg i.v. diphenhydramine 50 mg i.v.	metoclopramide 3 mg/kg i.v. 2 hourly × 1

Table 2. Assessment criteria

Emesis		Nausea	
Complete	no emetic episodes	None	
Major	1–2 emetic episodes	Mild	did not interfere with normal daily life
Minor	3–5 emetic episodes	Moderate	interfered with normal daily life
Failure	>5 emetic episodes	Severe	bedridden due to nausea

Table 3. Patient demography

	Ondansetron + dexamethasone	Metoclopramide + dexamethasone + diphenhydramine
Number of patients	145	142
Male	75	79
Female	70	63
Median age, years	60	60
Median dose of cisplatin, mg/m²	76	81

Introduction

Ondansetron, a highly selective 5-HT_3 receptor antagonist, is superior to high-dose metoclopramide in the control of acute emesis induced by high-dose cisplatin, one of the most emetogenic chemotherapeutic agents [1–3]. Ondansetron is also associated with a more favourable safety profile, since unlike metoclopramide, it does not induce extrapyramidal reactions via the direct antagonism of dopamine receptors. The addition of dexamethasone to ondansetron and metoclopramide enhances their efficacy [4–8]. Furthermore, the addition of diphenhydramine or lorazepam to regimens containing metoclopramide increases efficacy even further, and can be used to counter the side effects of metoclopramide [9, 10]. Prior to the introduction of the 5-HT_3 receptor antagonists, combinations such as metoclopramide plus dexamethasone and diphenhydramine or lorazepam were generally regarded as the most effective anti-emetic treatments for the control of emesis induced by high-dose cisplatin chemotherapy. This study was therefore conducted to compare one such regimen (metoclopramide plus dexamethasone and diphenhydramine) with ondansetron plus dexamethasone to determine the most effective anti-emetic therapy for cisplatin-induced emesis. The results of this study (in part) have previously been published [11].

Patients and Methods

This was a multicentre, randomised, double-blind, parallel group study, designed to recruit 284 adult patients scheduled to receive 1 or more courses of high-dose cisplatin (≥ 50 mg/m^2) chemotherapy. This sample size was determined in order to detect a 15% difference between the 2 regimens using 2-sided tests and a significance level of 5%. In a smaller sub-group of patients, it was possible to follow the effectiveness of the 2 regimens through a further 1 or 2 cycles of cisplatin chemotherapy.

Patients were excluded from the study if they had experienced emesis or received any other anti-emetics in the 24 h preceding cisplatin administration.

Anti-Emetic Dose Schedules

Patients were randomised to receive 1 of 2 intravenous anti-emetic regimens (table 1). Starting 47 min before cisplatin, diphenhydramine 50 mg or 2 ml of saline were given over 2 min followed immediately by 20 mg dexamethasone in 50 ml saline over 15 min. This was followed by a 15-min infusion of ondansetron (as ondansetron hydrochloride dihydrate) at a dose of 0.15 mg/kg or metoclopramide at a dose of 3 mg/kg diluted in 50 ml saline. After chemotherapy, 2 h after the first dose, the same dose of ondansetron or metoclopramide was administered. This was followed 2 h later by a further dose of ondansetron or 50 ml saline. In order to prevent cisplatin-induced delayed emesis, all patients received the same anti-emetic regimen of oral metoclopramide 20 mg every 6 h on days 2, 3 and 4. Patients were also given intramuscular dexamethasone 8 mg twice daily on days 2 and 3, and 4 mg twice daily on day 4.

Assessment

Nausea, emesis and adverse effects were recorded every 2 h for the first 8 h after cisplatin therapy and then daily for 4 days after cisplatin administration. These assessments were made in the hospital by the investigators for the first 24 h (acute emesis), and thereafter recorded daily on diary cards by the patients on an outpatient basis. Emesis and nausea were defined as described in table 2.

Results

Two hundred and eighty-nine patients were recruited into the study, 287 of these were evaluable according to the 'intention to treat' principle and 267 patients comprised the efficacy population (i.e. complied with the study protocol); 136 received the ondansetron regimen and 131 received the metoclopramide combination. The results presented here are for the efficacy population as the conclusions from the 'intention to treat' and efficacy populations did not differ. Patient characteristics were similar in the 2 groups (table 3).

Acute Emesis and Nausea

On day 1, ondansetron plus dexamethasone was significantly more effective than the metoclopramide combination in the control of acute emesis and nausea. Complete protection against emesis was achieved in 79% of patients given ondansetron plus dexamethasone as opposed to 59% given the metoclopramide combination ($p < 0.002$). Furthermore, major control was reported in an additional 15% of the ondansetron group and 25% of the metoclopramide group, giving a complete plus major control rate of 94% vs. 84% ($p < 0.02$), respectively. Complete protection against nausea was achieved in 77% of patients given ondansetron plus dexamethasone compared with 66% given the alternative regimen ($p < 0.051$). Complete success, i.e. no emesis and no nausea was also significantly superior in the ondansetron arm; 69% of the patients receiving ondansetron plus dexamethasone experienced no vomiting, retching or nausea compared with only 50% of those on the metoclopramide regimen ($p < 0.003$; fig. 1).

In those patients who did vomit or retch on the first day, the mean time to the first emetic episode was significantly longer in those patients given ondansetron plus dexamethasone (15.4 h) than in those given the metoclopramide combination (5.5 h). This difference was highly significant ($p < 0.0001$).

Delayed Emesis

For delayed emesis, protection was better on days 2 and 3 in those patients who had received ondansetron plus dexamethasone on day 1 than in those who had been treated with the metoclopramide combination (fig. 2). On day 4, the difference was not significant. Nausea was also better controlled on day 2 in patients receiving the ondansetron regimen; there were no significant differences on days 3 and 4 (fig. 3).

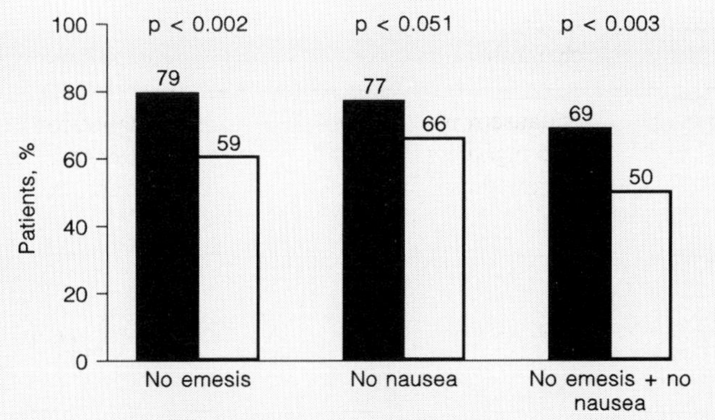

Fig. 1. Complete control of emesis and nausea on day 1. ■ = Ondansetron + dexamethasone; □ = metoclopramide + dexamethasone + diphenhydramine.

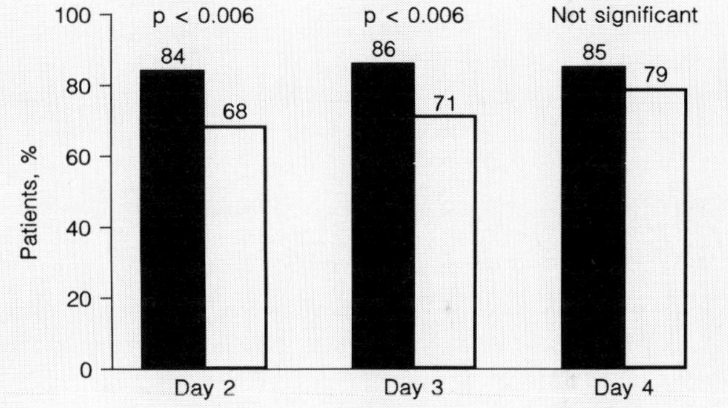

2

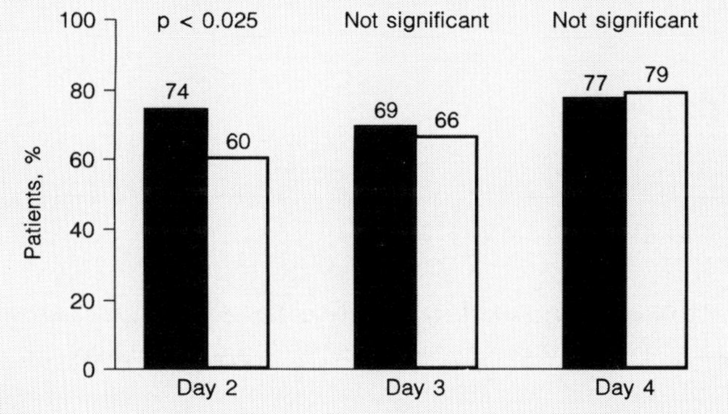

3

Fig. 2, 3. Complete control of delayed emesis (**2**) and nausea (**3**). Symbols are the same as in figure 1.

Table 4. Adverse events on day 1

	Ondansetron + dexamethasone n = 145	Metoclopramide + dexamethasone + diphenhydramine n = 144
Diarrhoea	2	7
Extrapyramidal reactions	0	4
Headache	4	2
Hot flush	3	0
Sedation	3	17*
Hiccup	2	1
Sweating	3	2
Other	9	23
Total	26	56**

* $p < 0.003$, ** $p < 0.0001$.

Subsequent Cycles

In those patients completing 2 and 3 cycles of cisplatin chemotherapy, the percentage of patients experiencing emesis in the metoclopramide group increased from 40 to 53%, but was almost constant in those given ondansetron plus dexamethasone.

Adverse Events

No severe or unexpected adverse effects were experienced by patients given either anti-emetic regimen. However, overall there were significantly fewer adverse events on day 1 in patients given ondansetron plus dexamethasone. Of the individual events, only sedation was significantly worse in the metoclopramide combination group and extrapyramidal reactions were only observed in metoclopramide-treated patients (3%; table 4).

Discussion

Despite the fact that regimens including high doses of metoclopramide are effective in reducing the incidence and severity of emesis and nausea during cisplatin chemotherapy, many patients still experience significant emesis [9, 10]. Unfortunately, it is not easy to make direct comparisons of the incidence of nausea and vomiting between studies carried out at different centres, or even between different studies carried out at the same centres, because of different prognostic factors in the study populations and differences in the cisplatin dosage regimens. However, it is possible to make comparisons within a study, provided that the patients and their treatments are themselves comparable. Although the protection afforded by ondansetron plus dexamethasone was lower in this study than in an earlier study conducted by our group [4], the patients in the two treatment groups described here were comparable, so it is reasonable to conclude that there was a real advantage with ondansetron plus dexamethasone over metoclopramide plus dexamethasone and diphenhydramine. Not only did ondansetron plus dexamethasone completely control acute emesis and nausea in more patients than did the metoclopramide combination, it also considerably delayed emesis in those patients who did eventually vomit on day 1. Moreover, overall tolerability was significantly superior with the ondansetron regimen, and as expected, it did not induce extrapyramidal reactions.

It is interesting that the advantage of ondansetron plus dexamethasone persisted to day 3 for emesis and to day 2 for nausea, despite the fact that ondansetron was given only on day 1. This indicates that good control on day 1 is carried over to good control on subsequent days. Perhaps even more important are the considerably better results with ondansetron plus dexamethasone in subsequent cisplatin treatment cycles. By the third cycle, 53% of patients given the metoclopramide combination were suffering acute emesis compared with only 26% of patients given the ondansetron regimen. This is very encouraging as it may allow chemotherapy to be given at undiminished doses for at least 3 cycles.

Conclusions

This study clearly demonstrates that combined therapy with ondansetron and dexamethasone is significantly more effective and better tolerated than metoclopramide plus dexamethasone and diphenhydramine for the prevention of cisplatin-induced emesis. The results of this study, therefore, suggest that ondansetron plus dexamethasone is ideally suited for preventing acute emesis and nausea following chemotherapy with high-dose cisplatin.

Appendix

Principal investigators: Medical Oncology Division, Policlinico Hospital, Perugia: F. Roila, MD, M. Tonato, MD; Medical Statistics Unit (Institute of Internal and Vascular Medicine), University of Perugia: E. Ballatori, PhD; Glaxo Group Research Limited, Middlesex, UK: D. Paes, MD; Institute of Internal Medicine I, University of Perugia, Italy: A. Del Favero, MD.

Statisticians: E. Ballatori, PhD, V. De Angelis, MD.

Investigators and collaborating centres: Medical Oncology Division, Perugia: C. Basurto, MD, S. Bracarda, MD, E. Corgna, MD, M. Picciafuoco, RN, L. Patoia, MD; Gynaecology Oncology Division, Brescia: G. Favalii, MD, R. Garbelli, MD, U.A. Bianchi, MD; Gynecology Oncology Division, Milano: G. Scarfone, MD, C. Ferraris, MD, M.C. Bolis, MD; Medical Oncology Division, Regina Elena Institute, Roma: F. Cognetti, MD, A. Cercato, MD; Medical Oncology Service, Terni: F. Buzzi, MD, S. Del Rio, MD; Medical Oncology Division, Modena: R. Sabbatini, MD, M. Federico, MD; Medical Oncology, University of Ancona: G. Matera, MD, R. Cellerino, MD; Medical Oncology Division, Ravenna: C. Dazzi, MD, M. Marangolo, MD; Medical Oncology Division, Piacenza: M. Leonardi, MD, R. Canaletti, MD; Gynecology Institute, Pavia: L. Babilonti, MD, C. Zara, MD; Medical Oncology Division, Ferrara: D. Donati, MD; Medical Oncology Division, Forli: D. Amadori, MD; Medical Oncology, Falck, Niguarda Hospital, Milano: M. Ferrari, MD.

References

1 De Mulder PHM, Seynaeve C, Vermorken JB, van Liessum PA, Mols-Jevdevic S, Lane Allman E, Beranek P, Verweij J: Ondansetron compared with high-dose metoclopramide in prophylaxis of acute and delayed cisplatin-induced nausea and vomiting. Ann Intern Med 1990;113:834–840.

2 Marty M, Pouillart P, Scholl S, Droz JP, Azab M, Brion N, Pujade-Lauraine E, Paule B, Paes D, Bons J: Comparison of the 5-hydroxytryptamine 3 (serotonin) antagonist ondansetron (GR 38032F) with high-dose metoclopramide in the control of cisplatin-induced emesis. N Engl J Med 1990;322:816–821.

3 Hainsworth J, Harvey W, Pendergrass K, Kasimis B, Oblon D, Monaghan G, Gandara D, Hesketh P, Khojasteh A, Harker G, York M, Siddiqui T, Finn A: A single-blind comparison of intravenous ondansetron, a selective serotonin antagonist, with intravenous metoclopramide in the prevention of nausea and vomiting associated with high-dose cisplatin chemotherapy. J Clin Oncol 1991;9:721–728.

4 Roila F, Tonato M, Cognetti F, Cortesi E, Favalli G, Marangolo M, Amadori D, Bella MA, Gramazio V, Donati D, Ballatori E, Del Favero A: Prevention of cisplatin-induced emesis: A double-blind multicentre randomised crossover study comparing ondansetron and ondansetron plus dexamethasone. J Clin Oncol 1991; 9:675–678.

5 Smyth JF, Coleman RE, Nicolson M, Gallmeier WM, Leonard RCF, Cornbleet MA, Allan SG, Upadhyaya BK, Bruntsch U: Does dexamethasone enhance control of acute cisplatin induced emesis by ondansetron? Br J Med 1991;303:1423–1426.

6 Smith DB, Newlands ES, Rustin GJS, Begent RHJ, Howells N, McQuade B, Bagshawe KD: Comparison of ondansetron and ondansetron plus dexamethasone as antiemetic prophylaxis during cisplatin-containing chemotherapy. Lancet 1991;338:487–490.

7 Roila F, Tonato M, Basurto C, Bella M, Passalacqua R, Morsia D, DiCostanzo F, Donati D, Ballatori E, Tognoni G, Del Favero A: Antiemetic activity of high doses of metoclopramide combined with methylprednisolone versus metoclopramide alone in cisplatin-treated cancer patients: A randomised double-blind trial of the Italian Oncology Group for Clinical Research. J Clin Oncol 1987;5:141–149.

8 Grunberg SM, Akerley WL, Krailo MD: Comparison of metoclopramide and metoclopramide plus dexamethasone for complete protection from cisplatin induced emesis. Cancer Invest 1986;4:379–385.

9 Kris MG, Gralla RJ, Clark RA, Tyson LB, Clark RA, Cirrincione C, Groshen S: Antiemetic control and prevention of side effects of anti-cancer therapy with lorazepam or diphenhydramine when used in combination with metoclopramide plus dexamethasone. Cancer 1987;60:2816–2822.

10 Roila F, Tonato M, Basurto C, Picciafuoco M, Bracarda S, Donati D, Malacarne P, Monici L, Di Costanzo F, Patoia L, Ballatori E, Tognoni G, Del Favero A: Protection from nausea and vomiting in cisplatin-treated patients: High-dose metoclopramide combined with methylprednisolone versus metoclopramide combined with dexamethasone and diphenhydramine: A study of the Italian oncology group for clinical research. J Clin Oncol 1989;7: 1693–1700.

11 Roila F, Italian Group for Antiemetic Research: Ondansetron + dexamethasone vs metoclopramide + dexamethasone + diphenhydramine in the prevention of cisplatin-induced emesis. Lancet 1992;340:96–99.

Oncology 1993;50:168–172

U. Räth[a]
B.K. Upadhyaya[b]
E. Arechavala[c]
H. Böckmann[d]
D. Dearnaley[e]
J.P. Droz[f]
S.D. Fosså[g]
R. Henriksson[h]
W.E. Aulitzky[i]
W.G. Jones[j]
L. Weissbach[k]
W. Paska[b]
A. Freeman[b]

[a] Klinikum der Universität Heidelberg, Heidelberg, FRG;
[b] Glaxo Group Research, Middlesex, UK;
[c] Hospital de Oncologia, Cuauhtémoc, Mexico;
[d] Rheinisch-Westfälische Technische Hochschule, Aachen, FRG;
[e] Royal Marsden Hospital, London, UK;
[f] Institut Gustave Roussy, Villejuif, France;
[g] Det Norske Radiumhospital, Oslo, Norway;
[h] Oncologkliniken, Umea, Sweden;
[i] Klinik der Universität, Mainz, FRG;
[j] Cookridge Hospital, Leeds, UK;
[k] Städtisches Krankenhaus, Berlin, FRG

Role of Ondansetron plus Dexamethasone in Fractionated Chemotherapy

Key Words
Ondansetron
Metoclopramide
Dexamethasone
Emesis
Fractionated chemotherapy

Abstract

This randomised, double-blind, parallel-group study was carried out to compare the efficacy and safety profile of ondansetron plus dexamethasone and metoclopramide plus dexamethasone in patients receiving fractionated cisplatin (20–25 mg/m^2/day) chemotherapy for the treatment of testicular cancer. An interim analysis of 95 patients showed that the ondansetron regimen was significantly superior compared to the metoclopramide regimen ($p < 0.001$). According to the study protocol the study was terminated at this stage. At the time the decision to stop the study was taken, a total of 113 patients had been enrolled and were evaluable on an 'intention to treat' basis. Fifty-six of these had received ondansetron (32 mg i.v. single dose/day) plus dexamethasone (20 mg i.v. single dose/day) and 57 were given metoclopramide (2 mg/kg or 1 mg/kg i.v. twice a day) plus dexamethasone (20 mg i.v. single dose/day). The ondansetron regimen was significantly superior in the control of emesis and nausea. Seventy-one percent of patients experienced 2 or fewer emetic episodes over the entire 5-day study period compared with 26% of patients given metoclopramide ($p < 0.001$). Seventy-nine percent of patients in the ondansetron group experienced 'none' or only 'mild' nausea compared with 39% of patients in the metoclopramide group ($p < 0.001$). The dose of metoclopramide had to be reduced during the study from 2 mg/kg i.v. twice daily to 1 mg/kg i.v. twice daily because 4 of the first 8 patients randomised to this treatment experienced extrapyramidal reactions. Ondansetron was well tolerated and it did not induce any extrapyramidal reactions. The results of this study show that ondansetron plus dexamethasone represents a very effective treatment option for patients receiving fractionated cisplatin chemotherapy for testicular cancer.

Introduction

Cisplatin is one of the most effective chemotherapeutic agents currently available. Its use in patients with testicular cancer results in cure rates of over 90% [1]. However, cisplatin is associated with a number of side effects such as nephrotoxicity and severe nausea and vomiting which are dose related. Cisplatin can be administered as a single dose (50–120 mg/m^2) or as a fractionated dose (20–40 mg/m^2/day) administered over a 4-or 5-day period. Frac-

Dr. U. Räth
Klinikum der Universität Heidelberg
Medizinische Klinik Abteilung IV
D-W–6900 Heidelberg (FRG)

tionated regimens are commonly used in the treatment of testicular cancer to maximise the tumour response and to reduce the side effects of treatment. Nevertheless, moderate to severe nausea and vomiting occurs in virtually all patients given such regimens if they are not adequately protected with anti-emetics [2]. Nausea and vomiting following chemotherapy can result in metabolic complications including dehydration, electrolyte imbalance, alkalosis and malnutrition. Moreover, the morbidity induced may lead to the premature termination of potentially curative chemotherapy.

None of the conventional anti-emetics such as high-dose metoclopramide are entirely effective in patients receiving cisplatin chemotherapy, although the efficacy of metoclopramide can be improved by the addition of dexamethasone [3–5]. However, the use of metoclopramide has been associated with a variety of side effects including extrapyramidal reactions and sedation. In particular, extrapyramidal symptoms are more frequent in younger patients (less than 30 years of age) [6] in whom testicular cancer is more common.

Ondansetron is a highly selective 5-HT_3 receptor antagonist and unlike metoclopramide will not induce extrapyramidal reactions via the direct antagonism of dopamine receptors. In single-dose cisplatin studies ondansetron is superior to high-dose metoclopramide [7, 8] and the addition of dexamethasone increases the efficacy of ondansetron [9, 10]. Indeed, a recent study has shown that ondansetron plus dexamethasone is superior to high-dose metoclopramide combined with dexamethasone and diphenhydramine [11]. Furthermore, a number of studies have demonstrated that ondansetron is effective when administered as a single intravenous dose (8–32 mg) before cisplatin chemotherapy [12–14].

Studies using ondansetron in fractionated cisplatin chemotherapy have reported good efficacy using a dose schedule of 0.15 mg/kg i.v. for 3 doses (total daily dose approximately 32 mg) [15, 16] and Sledge et al. [17] have shown that ondansetron is superior to high-dose metoclopramide. However, unlike the single-dose cisplatin studies, there have been no studies using a single-dose-per-day regimen of ondansetron and/or using a combination of ondansetron and dexamethasone.

This study was therefore carried out to determine the optimal anti-emetic treatment for patients receiving fractionated cisplatin chemotherapy for the treatment of testicular cancer. The efficacy and safety profile of ondansetron, given as a single dose, plus dexamethasone was compared with high-dose metoclopramide also given in combination with dexamethasone.

Patients and Methods

Conduct of the Study

The study was conducted in 10 centres in France, Germany, Mexico, Norway, Sweden and the United Kingdom according to Good Clinical Practice procedures and to the Declaration of Helsinki (1964) as modified by the 35th World Health Assembly, Venice, Italy (1983). The protocol received approval from local Ethics Committees, and consent was obtained from patients after an explanation of the study had been given.

Patients

Male patients aged at least 17 years with cancer of the testis due to receive their first daily course of chemotherapy and scheduled to receive a further 4 daily courses were included. The chemotherapy contained cisplatin (20–25 mg/m^2) either alone or in combination with other agents. Patients were excluded from the study if they had 1 or more of the following: severe concurrent illness, gastro-intestinal obstruction, central nervous system metastases, vomiting in the 24 h prior to chemotherapy, received anti-emetic therapy concurrently or in the 24 h before chemotherapy, or received benzodiazepines except when given for night sedation.

Study Design and Anti-Emetic Dose Schedules

This was a multicentre, randomised, double-blind parallel-group study designed to include 180 patients. The study was designed to detect a difference between success rates (0–2 emetic episodes over the 5 study days) of 60% with metoclopramide plus dexamethasone and 80% with ondansetron plus dexamethasone. Using 2-sided tests at an overall 5% significance level and a power of 0.8, 160 patients would be required. To ensure entry of 160 evaluable patients it was intended to recruit 180 patients. The study design allowed for an interim analysis of the results when the first 80 evaluable patients had completed the protocol. If the analysis of the primary efficacy response showed a significant difference between the 2 treatment regimens at the 5% level, the study would be terminated.

Patients were randomly assigned to receive 1 of 2 anti-emetic treatments (table 1). Ondansetron (as ondansetron hydrochloride dihydrate) at a dose of 32 mg or metoclopramide (2 or 1 mg/kg) were diluted to 100 ml in normal saline and administered as an intravenous infusion over 15 min, 30 min prior to cisplatin. Placebo infusion with normal saline or the same metoclopramide dose was repeated 90 min after the end of the cisplatin infusion. Patients in both treatment arms received dexamethasone at a dose of 20 mg (diluted to 10 ml in normal saline) as a slow intravenous injection immediately before the cisplatin infusion.

Assessment

The number and timing of vomits and retches, together with an assessment of nausea as none, mild, moderate or severe, were recorded daily by patients on diary cards. An emetic episode was defined as 1 vomit or retch (vomit, not productive of liquid). Emetic episodes were, by definition, separated by the absence of vomiting or retching for at least 1 min. The absence of emetic episodes was defined as complete control of emesis, 1 or 2 episodes as major control, 3–5 as minor control, and more than 5 as failure of the treatment. Patients achieving complete or major control were regarded as a success.

Table 1. The daily anti-emetic dose regimens used in the study

Treatment arm	Dose prior to cisplatin	Dose following cisplatin
A	ondansetron 32 mg i.v. dexamethasone 20 mg i.v.	placebo
B	metoclopramide 2 mg/kg[1] i.v. dexamethasone 20 mg i.v.	metoclopramide 2 mg/kg[1] i.v.

[1] The metoclopramide dose was reduced to 1 mg/kg during the study due to extrapyramidal reactions.

Table 2. Patient demography

		Ondansetron + dexamethasone	Metoclopramide + dexamethasone
Number of patients		56	57
Age, years	mean	32	32
	range	17–68	20–64
Weight, kg	mean	74.4	76.0
	range	46–111	47–108
Height, cm	mean	177	176
	range	156–194	154–194

Statistical Analyses

The total number of emetic episodes over all 5 days of treatment was analysed. The proportions of patients showing a complete (0 emetic episodes) and a complete or major response (0–2 emetic episodes) over the 5-day treatment period were compared between treatments using a 2-sided Mantel-Haenszel test. The total number of emetic episodes during the 5 days of treatment and the number of emesis-free days were compared between treatments using Wilcoxon's rank sum test. Patients who withdrew or received rescue medication were regarded as not emesis free from that day onwards.

The most severe grade of nausea on any study day was analysed. In addition, the proportions of days with nausea graded as 'none' or 'mild' were calculated for each patient and compared between treatments using Wilcoxon's rank sum test. Patients who withdrew or received rescue medication were regarded as failures with respect to nausea grade from that day onwards.

Adverse Events

Adverse events were reported as observed during the study with a further assessment 1–3 weeks after treatment. Routine haematological and biochemical assessments were carried out prior to the administration of the first dose of study drugs. Further blood samples were only required following the occurrence of clinically significant adverse events if thought appropriate by the investigator.

Results

An interim analysis was performed on a total of 95 patients of whom 47 had received ondansetron plus dexamethasone and 48 had received metoclopramide plus dexamethasone. At this stage the ondansetron regimen was found to be significantly superior when compared with the metoclopramide regimen; 66 and 27% of patients, respectively, had complete or major control of emesis (0–2 emetic episodes) over the entire 5-day treatment period ($p < 0.001$). Therefore, according to the study protocol, the study was terminated.

Following the termination of the study a total of 113 patients were evaluable on an 'intention to treat' basis (i.e. patients randomised to treatment and receiving at least 1 dose of cisplatin). Fifty-six of these patients received ondansetron plus dexamethasone and 57 received metoclopramide plus dexamethasone. The treatment groups were balanced with respect to age, weight and height (table 2). Analyses were performed on both the 'intention to treat' and the efficacy population (i.e. patients who fully complied with the study protocol). The results reviewed here are those for the 'intention to treat' population only, as there were no differences in the conclusions from the 2 sets of analyses.

Anti-Emetic Efficacy

On each of the 5 days of chemotherapy, control of emesis and nausea was superior with ondansetron plus dexamethasone compared with metoclopramide plus dexamethasone (fig. 1, 2). Comparing the total emetic response over the 5 days of chemotherapy, 71% of patients treated with the ondansetron regimen had complete or major control of emesis (0–2 emetic episodes) compared with 26% given the metoclopramide regimen ($p < 0.001$). Similarly, the control of nausea with the ondansetron regimen was significantly superior; 79% of patients in the ondansetron group experienced 'none' or 'mild' nausea over the 5 days of treatment compared with 39% of patients in the metoclopramide group ($p < 0.001$). The complete response rates (0 emetic episodes) over the 5 days of treatment were 57 and 19% for the ondansetron and metoclopramide groups, respectively ($p < 0.001$; fig. 3). Patients treated with ondansetron also had significantly fewer emetic episodes ($p < 0.001$) and significantly more emesis-free days ($p < 0.001$). The proportion of days with nausea graded as 'none' or 'mild' was also significantly greater for the ondansetron regimen ($p < 0.001$). Treatment with the metoclopramide regimen resulted in a significant proportion of patients requiring rescue medication and/or

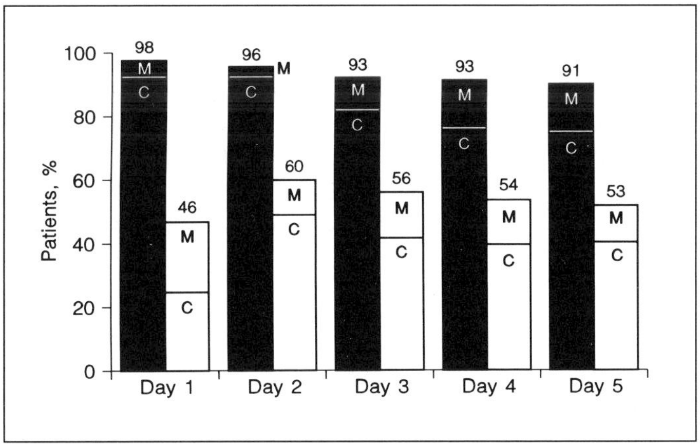

Fig. 1. Comparison of the anti-emetic effects of ondansetron plus dexamethasone (■) and metoclopramide plus dexamethasone (□) on each day of chemotherapy. C = Complete response; M = major response.

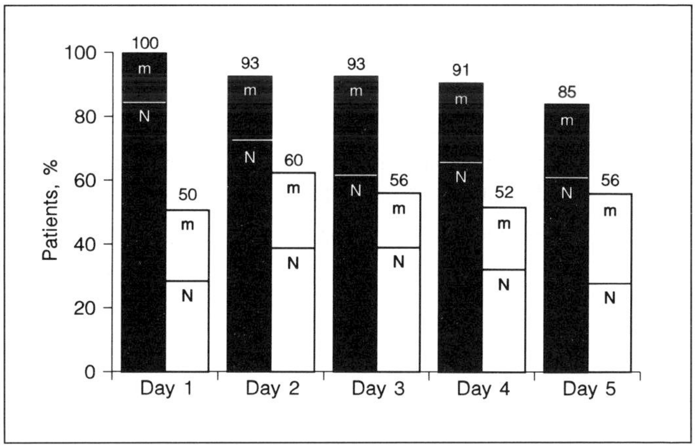

Fig. 2. Comparison of ondansetron plus dexamethsone (■) and metoclopramide plus dexamethasone (□) for the control of nausea on each day of chemotherapy. N = No nausea; m = mild nausea.

withdrawal from the study. Only 68% of patients on the metoclopramide regimen compared to 98% given the ondansetron regimen completed their course of chemotherapy on the same anti-emetic regimen.

Adverse Events

All 113 patients were included in the safety analysis. The dose of metoclopramide had to be reduced during the study from 2 mg/kg twice daily to 1 mg/kg twice daily because 4 of the first 8 patients randomised to this treatment experienced extrapyramidal symptoms. Of the 57 patients randomised to the metoclopramide regimen 10 (18%) patients received 2 mg/kg and 47 (82%) patients received 1 mg/kg. Seven out of 57 (12%) patients in the metoclopramide group had to withdraw from the study due to extrapyramidal symptoms. There were no extrapyramidal reactions in patients treated with ondansetron. Adverse events considered related to the ondansetron arm included constipation and headache which occurred in 5 and 4% of patients, respectively.

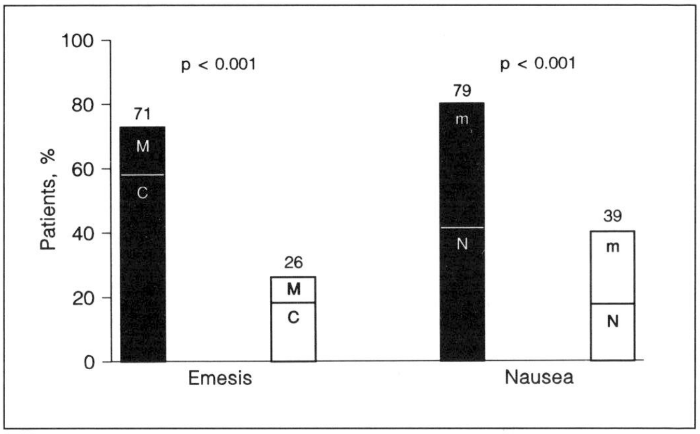

Fig. 3. Comparison of ondansetron plus dexamethasone (■) and metoclopramide plus dexamethasone (□) over days 1–5. C/N = Complete response/no nausea; M/m = major response/mild nausea.

Discussion

The results of this study have clearly shown that ondansetron plus dexamethasone is significantly superior to metoclopramide plus dexamethasone in patients receiving fractionated cisplatin chemotherapy for the treatment of testicular cancer. Seventy-one percent of patients treated with ondansetron compared with 26% given metoclopramide experienced 2 or fewer emetic episodes over the entire 5-day treatment period. Furthermore, none of the patients given ondansetron experienced extrapyramidal reactions. Metoclopramide is known to be associated with extrapyramidal reactions particularly in patients less than 30 years of age [6] in whom testicular cancer is more common. In this study, the dose of metoclopramide had to be reduced from 2 mg/kg twice daily to 1 mg/kg twice daily because 4 of the first 8 patients treated with metoclopramide experienced extrapyramidal symptoms. This lower dose of metoclopramide is within the dose range previously recommended for patients receiving cisplatin doses <40 mg/m^2 [18]. Diphenhydramine, which may have reduced the incidence of extrapyramidal reactions, was not used as it is not available in all the countries in which this study was conducted.

Nausea and vomiting are frequent and serious complications of cisplatin chemotherapy, affecting all patients who receive cisplatin daily for 5 days [2]. This may lead to serious complications and premature termination of potentially curative treatment. The results of this study show that ondansetron plus dexamethasone is an effective and well tolerated treatment option for fractionated cisplatin chemotherapy, particularly in patients under 30 years of age.

A single-dose regimen of 32 mg ondansetron was used in this study as it is now well established that single intravenous doses of ondansetron (8–32 mg) are effective in the control of acute emesis induced by cisplatin chemotherapy [12–14]. The selection of an appropriate dose (8–32 mg) is dependent on the emetogenic challenge and patient factor. For example, it is known that patients given higher doses of cisplatin will experience more emesis and that women are more susceptible than men to chemotherapy-induced emesis [18]. An 8 mg single-dose regimen of ondansetron may therefore be effective in male patients receiving low daily doses of cisplatin chemotherapy. This would enhance the cost-effectiveness of ondansetron although this requires further investigation.

Conclusions

This study has demonstrated that ondansetron plus dexamethasone is a significantly superior and better tolerated anti-emetic regimen than metoclopramide plus dexamethasone in patients receiving fractionated cisplatin chemotherapy for the treatment of testicular cancer. These results suggest that this combination (ondansetron plus dexamethasone) is ideally suited for this group of patients.

References

1 Einhorn LH: Complicated problems in testicular cancer. Semin Oncol 1988;15:9–15.

2 Einhorn LH, Williams SD: Combination chemotherapy with cis-diaminedichloroplatinum and adriamycin for testicular cancer refractory to vinblastine and bleomycin. Cancer Treat Rep 1978;62:1351–1353.

3 Allan SG, Cornbleet MA, Warrington PS, Golland IM, Leonard RCF, Smyth JF: Dexamethasone and high dose metoclopramide: Efficacy in controlling cisplatin induced nausea and vomiting. Br Med J 1984;289:878–879.

4 Rosell R, Abad-Esteve A, Ribas-Mundo M, Moreno I: Evaluation of a combination antiemetic regimen including iv high-dose metoclopramide, dexamethasone and diphenhydramine in cisplatin-based chemotherapy regimens. Cancer Treat Rep 1985;69:909–910.

5 Kris MG, Gralla RJ, Tyson LB, Clark RA, Kelsen DP, Reilly LK, Groshen S, Bosl GJ, Kalman LA: Improved control of cisplatin-induced emesis with high-dose metoclopramide and with combinations of metoclopramide, dexamethasone and diphenhydramine. Results of consecutive trials in 255 patients. Cancer 1985;55:527–534.

6 Kris MG, Tyson LB, Gralla RJ: Extrapyramidal reactions with high-dose metoclopramide. N Engl J Med 1983;309:433.

7 De Mulder PHM, Seynaeve C, Vermorken JB, van Liessum PA, Mols-Jevdevic S, Lane-Allman E, Beranek P, Verweij J: Ondansetron compared with high-dose metoclopramide in prophylaxis of acute and delayed cisplatin-induced nausea and vomiting. A multicentre, randomized, double-blind, crossover study. Ann Intern Med 1990;113:834–840.

8 Marty M, Pouillart P, Scholl S, Droz JP, Azab M, Brion N, Pujade-Lauraine E, Paule B, Paes D, Bons J: Comparison of the 5-hydroxytryptamine 3 (serotonin) antagonist ondansetron (GR38032F) with high dose metoclopramide in the control of cisplatin-induced emesis. N Engl J Med 1990;322:816–821.

9 Roila F, Tonato M, Cognetti F, Cortesi E, Favalli G, Marangolo M, Amadori D, Bella MA, Gramazio V, Donati D, Ballatri E, Del Favero A: Prevention of cisplatin-induced emesis: A double-blind multicentre randomised crossover study comparing ondansetron and ondansetron plus dexamethasone. J Clin Oncol 1991; 9:675–678.

10 Smyth JF, Coleman RE, Nicolson M, Gallmeier WM, Leonard RCF, Cornbleet MA, Allan SG, Upadhyaya BK, Bruntsch U: Does dexamethasone enhance control of acute cisplatin-induced emesis by ondansetron? Br Med J 1991;303:1423–1426.

11 Roila F, Italian Group for Antiemetic Research: Ondansetron + dexamethasone vs metoclopramide + dexamethasone + diphenhydramine in prevention of cisplatin-induced emesis. Lancet 1992;340:96–99.

12 Seynaeve C, Schuller J, Buser K, Porteder H, Van Belle S, Sevelda P, Christmann D, Schmidt M, Kitchener H, Paes D, de Mulder PHM: Comparison of the anti-emetic efficacy of different doses of ondansetron, given as either a continuous infusion or a single intravenous dose, in acute cisplatin-induced emesis. A multicentre, double-blind, randomised, parallel group study. Br J Cancer 1992;66:192–197.

13 Marty M, d'Allens H: Double-blind multicentre study of 2 dose schedules of intravenous ondansetron in the control of cisplatin-induced emesis: Single dose vs continuous infusion. Cah Cancer 1990;2:541–546.

14 Beck TM, Hesketh PJ, Madajewicz S, Navari RM, Pendergrass K, Lester EP, Kish JA, Murphy WK, Hainsworth JD, Gandara DR, Bricker LJ, Keller AM, Mortimer J, Galvin DV, House KW, Bryson JC: Stratified, randomised, double-blind comparison of intravenous ondansetron administered as a multiple-dose regimen versus two single-dose regimens in the prevention of cisplatin-induced nausea and vomiting. J Clin Oncol 1992;10:1969–1975.

15 Einhorn LH, Nagy C, Werner K, Finn AL: Ondansetron: A new effective antiemetic for patients receiving cisplatin chemotherapy. J Clin Oncol 1990;8:731–735.

16 Burton G, Huang A, Lazarus H, Moore J, House KW, Finn AL: A double-blind randomized comparison of three doses of i.v. ondansetron for prevention of emesis induced by multiday cisplatin chemotherapy (abstract). Proc Am Soc Clin Oncol 1990;9:1269.

17 Sledge GW, Einhorn LH, Nagy C, House K: Phase III double-blind comparison of intravenous ondansetron and metoclopramide as antiemetic therapy for patients receiving multiple-day cisplatin-based chemotherapy. Cancer 1992;70:2524–2528.

18 Gralla, RJ: An outline anti-emetic treatment. Eur J Cancer Clin Oncol 1989;25(suppl 1):S7–S11.

Oncology 1993;50:173–179

J.T. Roberts[a]
T.J. Priestman[b]

[a] Regional Radiotherapy Centre, Newcastle General Hospital, Newcastle upon Tyne;
[b] The Royal Hospital, Wolverhampton, UK

A Review of Ondansetron in the Management of Radiotherapy-Induced Emesis

Key Words
Ondansetron
Metoclopramide
Prochlorperazine
Radiotherapy
Emesis
Total body irradiation

Abstract
This paper reviews experience with ondansetron in radiotherapy-induced emesis. The efficacy of ondansetron is assessed following a number of different radiotherapy regimens: single-dose radiotherapy, fractionated radiotherapy, total body irradiation (TBI) and hemi-body irradiation. In single-dose radiation-induced emesis, ondansetron (8 mg orally 3 times daily) provided superior anti-emetic control compared with metoclopramide (10 mg orally 3 times daily): 92 and 46% of patients, respectively, experienced complete control of emesis (0 emetic episodes) in the first 24 h following treatment ($p < 0.001$). Similarly, ondansetron (8 mg orally 3 times daily) was significantly ($p < 0.001$) more effective than prochlorperazine (10 mg orally 3 times daily) with 59 and 35% of patients, respectively, achieving complete control of emesis on the 'worst day' of a fractionated radiotherapy regimen (up to 20 fractions). Two studies evaluating the efficacy of ondansetron in TBI-induced emesis have demonstrated that ondansetron is effective in paediatric and adult patients receiving chemotherapy and TBI prior to bone marrow transplantation. In these studies, 57–81% of patients experienced 2 or fewer emetic episodes during TBI. For hemi-body irradiation, ondansetron (8 mg) and dexamethasone (8 mg) given orally produced complete control of emesis in 12 out of 14 patients. The effectiveness of this regimen now enables patients receiving hemi-body irradiation to be treated as outpatients in many cases. Anecdotal data also shows that ondansetron is effective when given as intervention treatment in patients with established emesis. In none of the studies were there any serious adverse events following ondansetron treatment. It can therefore be concluded that ondansetron is an effective and well tolerated anti-emetic for the prophylaxis and treatment of radiation-induced emesis and nausea. The use of effective anti-emetic treatments may have resource implications such as reducing bed occupancy and enabling the use of fewer, larger fractions of radiotherapy.

Presented on behalf of the Ondansetron Radiotherapy Study Group (see Appendix for details).

J.T. Roberts
Regional Radiotherapy Centre
Newcastle General Hospital
Westgate Road
Newcastle upon Tyne NE4 6BE (UK)

Introduction

A substantial minority of patients receiving radiotherapy will experience distressing nausea and vomiting. The degree of emesis will vary but is generally less severe than that associated with cisplatin-based chemotherapy. However, since a course of radiation may involve up to 30 or 40 fractions given over a period of 6–8 weeks, the potential for distress to the patient due to sickness continuing for that length of time is considerable. There is a small body of literature on the use of conventional anti-emetics (metoclopramide, prochlorperazine, chlorpromazine, domperidone and nabilone) in the prevention or treatment of radiation-induced emesis. These agents appear to be effective in approximately 50% of patients. This paper reviews the factors that influence the incidence and severity of radiotherapy-induced emesis and clinical trial results using ondansetron (as ondansetron hydrochloride dihydrate) in this setting.

Factors that Influence the Incidence and Severity of Radiotherapy-Induced Emesis

The pathophysiology of radiation-induced emesis remains incompletely understood but a number of factors which predict the likelihood of radiation-induced emesis have been identified.

Site

Radiotherapy to the upper abdomen is most likely to produce emesis and nausea. Animal studies have shown that such irradiation causes the release of emetic substances from the first part of the small bowel. Stimulation of the chemoreceptor trigger zone via vagal afferent fibres from the upper gastrointestinal tract has also been implicated [1]. Although theoretical pathways exist to explain the mechanism by which upper abdominal irradiation causes emesis, it remains the case that a small but significant proportion of patients receiving radiotherapy to other sites may experience considerable emesis.

Field Size

The greater the volume of tissue irradiated, the greater the risk of emesis and nausea. Total body irradiation (TBI) therefore presents the greatest emetic challenge.

Dose per Fraction

The greater the dose of radiation given at each treatment, the greater the risk of emesis. Palliative radiotherapy may be given with single exposures of 8–15 Gy, greatly increasing the risk of emesis for these patients. Patients receiving more than 8 Gy as a single dose are more likely to experience emesis than those patients receiving smaller doses of approximately 2 Gy as in fractionated radiotherapy. However, there is also evidence to suggest that emesis occurs following a cumulative dosing threshold of >3 Gy [2].

Age

Compared with the effects of chemotherapy, where children are more likely to experience emesis, there is some evidence to suggest that children are less susceptible to radiation-induced emesis than adults, particularly during TBI.

Anxiety

As with chemotherapy, there are suggestions that anxiety and apprehension may increase the likelihood of sickness in patients receiving radiotherapy.

Effect of Ondansetron against Radiation-Induced Emesis

Efficacy of Ondansetron against Single-Dose Radiotherapy-Induced Emesis

A study has been done to compare the efficacy and safety profile of ondansetron and metoclopramide following single-dose radiotherapy to the upper abdomen [3].

Patients and Methods

This was a randomised, double-blind, parallel group study. Patients were scheduled to receive single, high-dose radiotherapy to the upper abdomen. Radiation doses of 8–10 Gy were given to fields of either 80–100 cm^2 centred between T10 and L2 inclusive or fields of 100–150 cm^2 centred between T8 and L3. Patients were randomised to receive either ondansetron (8 mg) or metoclopramide (10 mg) orally 3 times daily. The initial anti-emetic dose was given 1–2 h prior to radiotherapy and continued for 3–5 days after the initiation of radiotherapy. Diary cards were used to record daily the incidence and severity of nausea and emesis. Nausea was graded as none, mild (did not interfere with normal daily life), moderate (interfered with normal daily life) or severe (bedridden due to nausea). An emetic episode was defined as any episode of vomiting or retching, with a minimum interval of 1 min between separate episodes. Responses were categorised as follows: complete (0 emetic episodes in 24 h), major (1–2 emetic episodes), minor (3–5 emetic episodes) and failure (>5 emetic episodes or administration of rescue anti-emetic treatment).

Results

One hundred and twenty-one patients (median age 63 years, range 33–83 years; 57 male, 64 female) entered the study of whom 105 were evaluable. The results showed a highly significant difference in efficacy in favour of ondansetron for the control of emesis ($p < 0.001$; fig. 1). Ninety-two percent of patients receiving ondansetron had complete control of emesis (0 emetic episodes) in the first 24 h, and in the remaining 8% there was major control of emesis (1–2 emetic episodes). In contrast, only 46% of patients receiving metoclopramide had complete control of emesis; major control was achieved in a further 25%, but 28% failed to be controlled or achieved only minor control ($\geqslant 3$ emetic episodes). With regard to nausea, 88% of patients receiving ondansetron had 'none' or 'mild' nausea compared to 60% of those receiving metoclopramide. Only 2% of ondansetron-treated patients experienced severe nausea, while nausea failed to be controlled in 21% of metoclopramide-treated patients. Overall, control of nausea was significantly greater in the ondansetron group ($p < 0.001$). Ondansetron continued to provide good control of emesis over the 5 days of the study with 98–100% of patients achieving a complete or major response over days 2–5 compared with 86–96% of patients receiving metoclopramide. The difference in efficacy between the 2 treatment groups, however, was not statistically significant, which may be related to the reduced emetic effect of the radiation dose over days 2–5. Nausea continued to be controlled in approximately 75–85% of patients in each group.

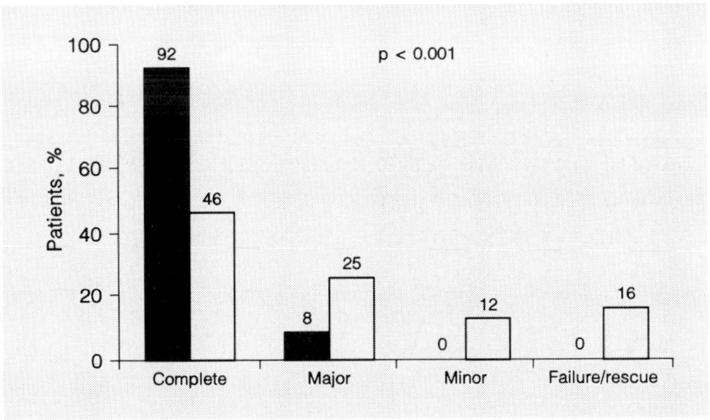

Fig. 1. Comparison of ondansetron (■, n =49) and metoclopramide (□, n = 56) following single high-dose radiotherapy.

Table 1. Characteristics of patients receiving fractionated radiotherapy

	Ondansetron	Prochlorperazine
Number of patients	98	94
Gender, male/female	60/38	58/36
Age, years		
median	57	63
range	26–85	21–84
Radiotherapy fractions		
<5[1]	2	11
5	33	39
>5	63	44

1 Due to anti-emetic treatment failure or withdrawal.

Efficacy of Ondansetron against Fractionated Radiotherapy-Induced Emesis

A study has been conducted comparing the efficacy of ondansetron and prochlorperazine in patients receiving fractionated dose regimens of radiotherapy [4].

Patients and Methods

This was a prospective, randomised, double-blind, multicentre comparative study. All patients were scheduled to receive a course of fractionated irradiation to the upper abdomen, consisting of 5 or more daily treatments (to a maximum of 20) with fractionated doses of 1.8 Gy or more to opposed single anterior or posterior fields to an area ≥ 100 cm^2 between the upper border of T11 and the lower border of L3. Patients were randomised to receive either ondansetron (8 mg) or prochlorperazine (10 mg) orally 3 times daily. Anti-emetic treatment commenced 1–2 hours before the first radiotherapy fraction and was continued for up to 3 days after the end of the radiotherapy course. The incidence of emesis (defined as previously described in this review) and the severity of nausea were recorded daily by the patients on diary cards.

Results

A total of 192 patients with malignant disease, aged at least 18 years, were entered into the study. Patient characteristics were similar between the 2 treatment groups (table 1). Ondansetron was significantly superior to prochlorperazine (fig. 2). On the 'worst day' for emesis of the fractionated radiotherapy treatment 59% of patients receiving ondansetron had a complete response (0 emetic episodes) compared with 35% given prochlorperazine ($p < 0.001$). When emesis control was evaluated according to the number of fractions of radiotherapy received, ondansetron provided complete control in a greater proportion of patients than prochlorperazine irrespective of the length of fractionated treatment (fig. 3). Furthermore, a significantly greater proportion of emesis-free days were

2 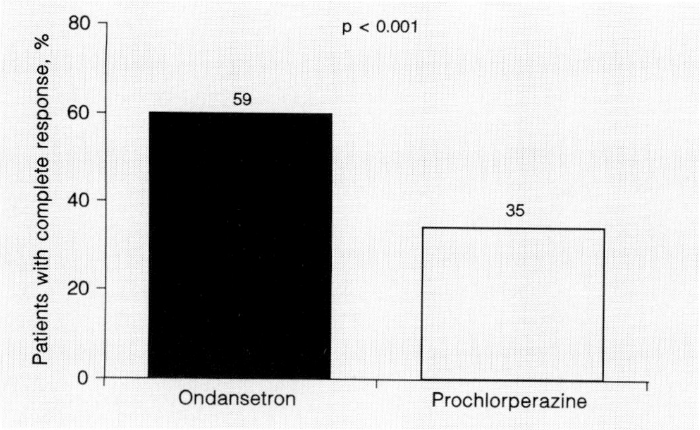

3 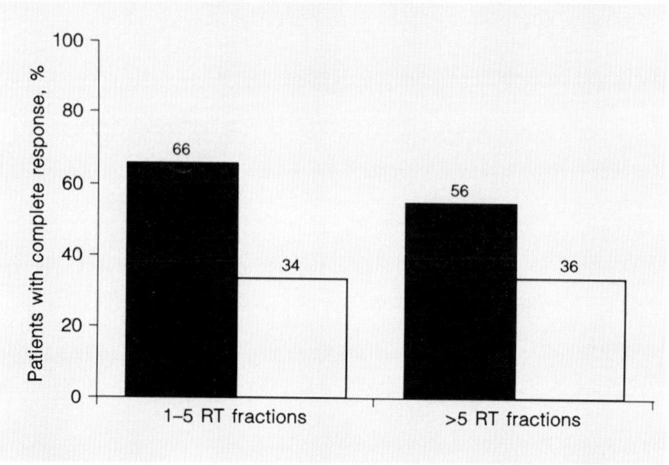

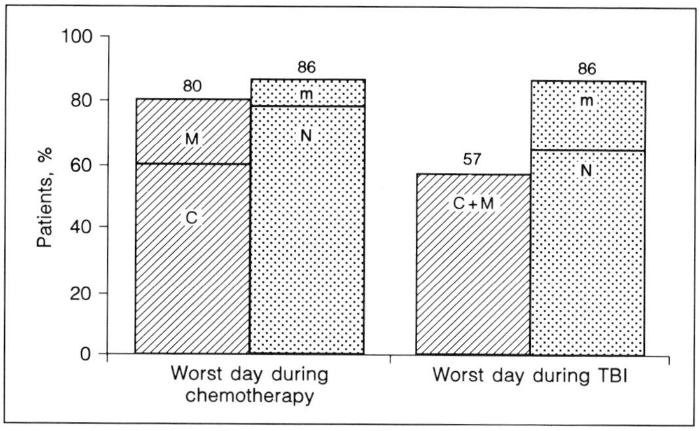 4

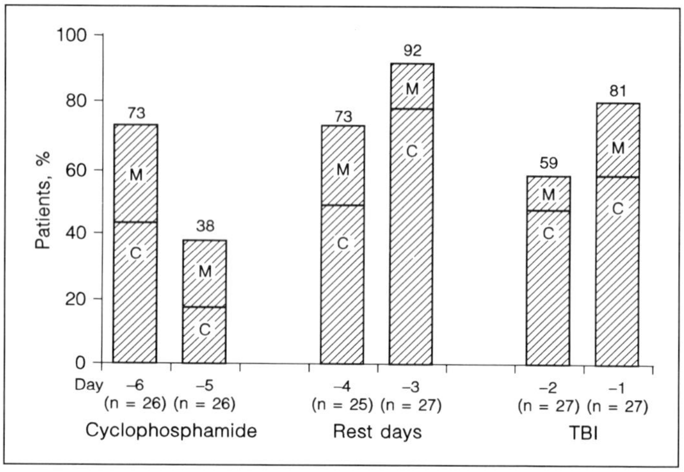 5

Fig. 2. Comparison of ondansetron (■) (n = 98) and prochlorperazine (□) (n = 94) in the control of fractionated radiotherapy-induced emesis, 'worst day' analysis.

Fig. 3. Comparison of ondansetron (■) and prochlorperazine (□) in the control of fractionated radiotherapy (RT) induced emesis by number of fractions.

Fig. 4. Efficacy of ondansetron in children during conditioning for BMT (study 1). ▨ = Emesis; ▩ = nausea; C/N = complete response/no nausea; M/m = major response/mild nausea.

Fig. 5. Control of emesis during conditioning for BMT (study 2). C = Complete response; M = major response.

observed in the ondansetron-treated patients (59%) than in those receiving prochlorperazine (39%) ($p = 0.05$). Nausea, however, was controlled equally well by both anti-emetics.

Efficacy of Ondansetron against TBI-Induced Emesis

Despite the use of conventional anti-emetics such as metoclopramide, emesis and nausea are almost universal after TBI and are equally prevalent whether treatment is given as a single dose or in a fractionated course with doses as low as 1.2 Gy daily [2]. Two open pilot studies have examined the use of ondansetron in children and adults undergoing conditioning prior to bone marrow transplantation (BMT) [6, 7]. Conditioning included both chemotherapy (high-dose cyclophosphamide) and TBI, which are extremely emetogenic. Separate assessments of emesis control were made for the 2 components of the conditioning process.

Patients and Methods

Study 1 included children whose ages ranged from 2 to 17 years and study 2 included patients with an age range of 13–51 years. Both groups of patients were scheduled to receive conditioning chemotherapy and TBI prior to BMT. The treatment regimens (TBI, chemotherapy and anti-emetic) for both studies are shown in table 2. In the paediatric study (study 1), the dose of ondansetron administered was based on the surface area of the child. Patients (or nurses) recorded daily on diary cards the occurrence of any nausea (graded as none, mild, moderate or severe) and emetic episodes (vomiting or retching) throughout the conditioning periods. Control of emesis as

Table 2. Conditioning and anti-emetic regimens

Treatment	Study 1	Study 2
Chemotherapy	*Leukaemia (n = 14)* cyclophosphamide 60 mg/kg on 2 consecutive days (days –6 and –5) followed by 1 day rest (day 4)	cyclophosphamide 60 mg/kg on 2 consecutive days (days –6 and –5) followed by 2 days rest (days –4 and –3)
	Aplastic anaemia (n = 1) cyclophosphamide 50 mg/kg for 4 consective days	
TBI	1.8 Gy twice daily for 4 consecutive days prior to BMT (days –3 to 0)	6 Gy as a single dose on 2 consecutive days (days –2 and –1) prior to BMT (day 0)
Ondansetron dose	*$SA < 1.2\ m^2$* $5\ mg/m^2$ i.v. three times daily during conditioning followed by 4 mg (2 mg if $SA < 0.6\ m^2$) orally three times daily for 2 days after BMT	8 mg i.v. three times daily during conditioning and for up to 7 days after BMT
	$SA > 1.2\ m^2$ 8 mg (maximum) i.v. three times daily followed by 8 mg orally three times daily for 2 days after BMT	

SA = Surface area.

complete, major, minor and failure were defined as previously described. The patients were reviewed daily for evidence of adverse effects.

Results

Fifteen patients were recruited into study 1. Study 2 included 30 patients of whom 16–27 were evaluable on each day. In study 1, complete or major control of emesis (0–2 emetic episodes) was achieved in 80 and 57% of patients during the 'worst day' of conditioning chemotherapy and TBI, respectively. Nausea was also well controlled during the 2 phases of treatment (fig. 4). In study 2, 59 and 81% of patients had complete or major control of emesis during the first and second day of TBI, respectively (fig. 5). Complete or major control was maintained in 75–82% of patients after BMT.

Efficacy of Ondansetron plus Dexamethasone against Hemi-Body Irradiation-Induced Emesis

Patients and Methods

In a pilot study at the Regional Radiotherapy Centre in Newcastle, the effects of premedication with a combination of ondansetron (8 mg) and dexamethasone (8 mg) were studied. Both anti-emetics were given orally, approximately 1 h before hemi-body irradiation for the palliation of bone pain from metastatic prostate cancer.

Results

Eleven men aged between 57 and 78 years received 14 doses of hemi-body irradiation. In 13 cases, 8 Gy was given as a single fraction to the lower half body, and in one case 6 Gy to the upper half body. During the first 24 h following radiotherapy, complete control of emesis was achieved in 12 of 14 (86%) cases. One patient experienced moderate and another mild nausea during the first 24 h. Nausea, with or without vomiting, became apparent 27–72 h after the single dose of radiation in 6 patients.

Since this regimen has proved to be effective, patients receiving hemi-body irradiation are now often treated in this unit as outpatients. This therefore has economic implications, since patients were previously admitted to hospital for 2 nights in order to control nausea and vomiting.

Efficacy of Ondansetron as Intervention Therapy against Established Radiation-Induced Emesis

Clinical trials have concentrated on the prophylactic use of ondansetron for the control of emesis and nausea associated with radiotherapy. However, clinical experience would indicate that, as in the ferret, ondansetron is also effective in reducing or abolishing established radio-

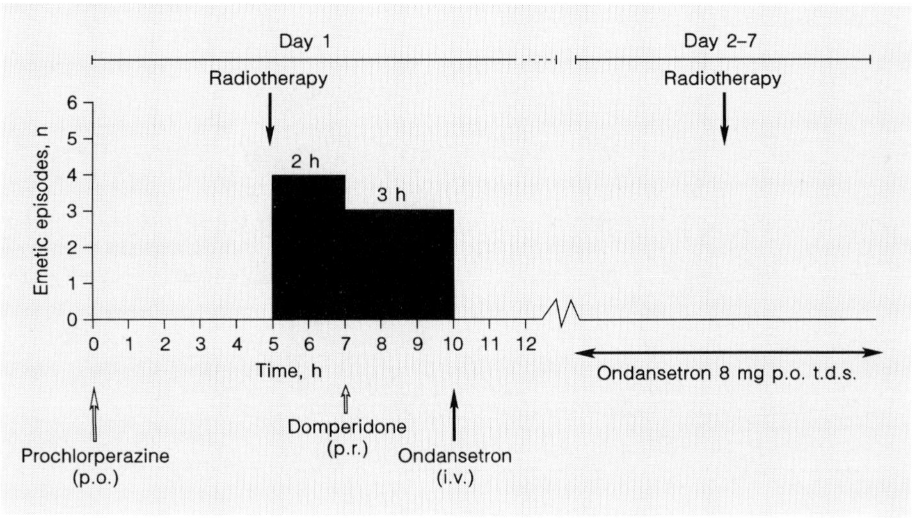

Fig. 6. Case study showing abolition of radiation-induced nausea and emesis with ondansetron.

therapy-induced nausea and vomiting. Experience in patients receiving fractionated abdominal irradiation suggests that ondansetron is also effective in refractory emesis following radiotherapy [8]. This is illustrated by the following case.

Case Study

A 63-year-old man with bone metastases from lung cancer experienced nausea before treatment, despite regular use of prochlorperazine. He received radiotherapy to the lumbar spine which produced emesis almost immediately, with 4 episodes of emesis in the first 2 h following radiotherapy. A domperidone (30 mg) suppository failed to stop the emesis (fig. 6). However, a single intravenous dose of ondansetron (8 mg) abolished emesis immediately. The patient therefore received regular oral doses of ondansetron and was able to continue his palliative course of radiotherapy with no further ill effects.

Adverse Events

Few adverse effects have been observed with the use of ondansetron in radiation-induced emesis. In the studies reviewed here, constipation was more common in patients receiving fractionated radiotherapy [3], especially those patients who had received ondansetron for a number of weeks, but this was not severe.

Discussion

Ondansetron has been shown to be an effective and well-tolerated anti-emetic for the control of emesis and nausea produced by a number of radiotherapy regimens: (1) single, high-dose radiotherapy; (2) fractionated radiotherapy; (3) TBI (in adults and children); (4) hemi-body radiotherapy (in combination with dexamethasone).

In single-dose and fractionated radiotherapy, ondansetron has been shown to be significantly superior to metoclopramide and prochlorperazine, respectively. For TBI and hemi-body irradiation non-comparative pilot studies have reported good efficacy for ondansetron administered alone and in combination with dexamethasone, respectively. In addition, anecdotal data has shown that ondansetron is effective when given to treat established emesis; ondansetron is therefore also a useful rescue medication should other agents fail as first-line therapy.

The effectiveness of ondansetron should reduce the morbidity of radiotherapy treatment particularly that associated with fractionated radiotherapy which may be given over a number of weeks. The use of an effective anti-emetic such as ondansetron may also enable radiotherapy to be administered on an outpatient basis, thereby reducing bed occupancy. Indeed, routine prophylaxis with ondansetron should allow the use of fewer, larger fractions of radiation for the palliation of, for example, lumbar spine metastases with the virtual certainty that the patient will escape the distressing sequelae of emesis and nausea. This in turn should mean fewer visits to a Radiotherapy Department for patients with incurable malignancies and allow the more efficient use of scarce and expensive radiotherapy equipment.

Conclusions

Ondansetron is an effective and well tolerated anti-emetic in the prophylaxis and treatment of radiotherapy-induced emesis. The use of an effective anti-emetic treatment such as ondansetron may have resource implications, reducing bed occupancy and enabling the use of fewer, larger fractions of radiotherapy.

Appendix

The Ondansetron Radiotherapy study group contributed to 3 studies described in this review. These studies were coordinated by B. Upadhyaya, Glaxo Group Research Limited, Middlesex, UK.

United Kingdom: W.P. Abram, M. Adams, C. Collis, M. Hewitt, F.G.C. Jones, H. Lucraft, A.J. Slater;
Eire: M. Moriarty;
Finland: M.S. Almo;
New Zealand: A.S. Abdelaal, D. Lamb;
The Netherlands: T. De Witte, S. Croockewit.

References

1 Harding RK: Prodromal effects of radiation: Pathway models and protection by anti-emetics. Pharmacol Ther 1988;39:335–345.
2 Westbrook C, Glaholm J, Barrett A: Vomiting associated with whole body irradiation. Clin Radiol 1987;38:263–266.
3 Collis CH, Priestman TJ, Priestman S, Lucraft H, Roberts JT, Adams M, Upadhyaya BK: The final assessment of a randomised double-blind comparative study of ondansetron vs. metoclopramide in the prevention of nausea and vomiting following high-dose upper abdominal irradiation. Clin Oncol 1991;3:241–242.
4 Priestman TJ, Roberts JT, Upadhyaya BK: Randomised, double-blind trial of ondansetron (OND) and prochlorperazine (PCP) in the prevention of fractionated radiotherapy (RT) induced emesis. Proc Am Soc Clin Oncol 1992;9: abstract 1370.
5 Franzén L, Israelsson G, Lomberg H, Modig H, Henriksson R: Ondansetron prevents emesis induced by fractionated radiotherapy. Eur J Cancer 1991;2 (suppl):S295, abstract 1807.
6 Jurgens H, McQuade B: Ondansetron as prophylaxis for chemotherapy and radiotherapy-induced emesis in children. Oncology 1992;49: 279–285.
7 Hewitt M, Croockewit S, Abram WP, Upadhyaya BK, Lane-Allman E: Ondansetron prophylaxis against emesis produced by total body irradiation and chemotherapy conditioning for bone marrow transplantation (abstract). Eur J Cancer 1991;2 (suppl):2949, abstract 1087.
8 Roberts JT: Ondansetron in the control of refractory emesis following radiotherapy. Clin Oncol 1992;4:67–68.

Oncology 1993;50:180–185

M. Clavel[a]
M. Soukop[b]
Y.L.A. Greenstreet[c]

[a] Centre Régional Léon Berard, Lyon, France;
[b] Royal Infirmary, Glasgow;
[c] Glaxo Group Research, Stockley Park, Uxbridge, UK

Improved Control of Emesis and Quality of Life with Ondansetron in Breast Cancer

Key Words
Ondansetron
Metoclopramide
Alizapride
Quality of life
Cyclophosphamide
Breast cancer

Abstract
Cyclophosphamide-based chemotherapy is often given to patients for the treatment of breast cancer. This chemotherapy can induce severe nausea and vomiting in these patients, which can adversely affect their quality of life, especially as these regimens are often given on an outpatient basis over several courses. This paper reviews 5 randomised, double-blind, multicentre comparative studies which have been carried out in breast cancer patients to evaluate the efficacy and safety profile of the potent and highly selective 5-HT_3 receptor antagonist, ondansetron. These studies have shown that ondansetron is superior to placebo in the control of emesis induced by a 14-day CMF schedule and that it is superior to conventional anti-emetics (metoclopramide and alizapride) in the control of acute and delayed emesis induced by regimens containing high-dose cyclophosphamide. Ondansetron was well tolerated in these studies and did not induce any extrapyramidal reactions. The efficacy and tolerability of ondansetron was reflected in a better quality of life for patients given this anti-emetic which was formally assessed in 2 of the studies using the Rotterdam Symptom Checklist or the Functional Living Index – Emesis. In conclusion, ondansetron is an effective and well-tolerated anti-emetic for patients receiving cyclophosphamide-based chemotherapy for the treatment of breast cancer. Ondansetron provides significant benefits for patients' quality of life compared with conventional anti-emetics particularly as these patients are often treated on an outpatient basis and can be treated with oral ondansetron at home.

Introduction

Breast cancer is the most common neoplasm affecting women in Western Europe and North America with an incidence of 1 in 10. Chemotherapy with regimens containing cyclophosphamide, sometimes together with doxorubicin or epirubicin, are effective in reducing recurrence rates and extending survival in patients with early or advanced disease [1]. This chemotherapy is usually given over several courses on an outpatient basis and can induce nausea and vomiting in over 80% of patients [2–4]. These symptoms can persist for several days after chemotherapy and may cause patients to refuse further courses of potentially curative therapy. Ondansetron is a

M. Clavel
Centre Régional Léon Berard
F–69000 Lyon (France)

Table 1. Design of studies with ondansetron in breast cancer patients

Study	Design	Chemotherapy	Ondansetron	Comparator
1	Parallel group	CMF (14 days)	8 mg orally before chemotherapy followed by 8 mg orally 3 times daily for 15 days	placebo orally before chemotherapy followed by oral dosing 3 times daily for 15 days
2	Cross-over	FAC/FEC	8 mg before chemotherapy (4 mg p.o., 4 mg i.v.) followed by 8 mg orally 3 times daily for 3–5 days	metoclopramide 80 mg (20 mg p.o., 60 mg i.v.) followed by 20 mg orally 3 times daily for 3–5 days
3	Parallel group	EC	8 mg orally before chemotherapy followed by 8 mg orally 3 times daily for 3–5 days	metoclopramide 60 mg i.v. before chemotherapy followed by 20 mg orally 3 times daily for 3–5 days
4	Parallel group	CMF/FAC/FEC	8 mg i.v. plus dexamethasone 16 mg i.v. before chemotherapy followed by 8 mg orally 3 times daily for 5 days	metoclopramide 60 mg i.v. plus dexamethasone 16 mg i.v. before chemotherapy followed by metoclopramide 20 mg orally 3 times a day for 5 days
5	Parallel group	FAC/FEC	8 mg orally before chemotherapy followed by 8 mg orally twice daily for 3–5 days	alizapride 150 mg i.v. before chemotherapy followed by 50 mg orally twice daily for 3–5 days.

C = Cyclophosphamide; A = doxorubicin; F = 5-fluorouracil; E = epirubicin; M = methotrexate.

potent and highly selective 5-HT_3 receptor antagonist which achieves complete or major control of emesis in 70–80% of patients treated with cisplatin- or cyclophosphamide-based chemotherapy regimens [5, 6], with further improvements in efficacy following the addition of dexamethasone [7, 8]. This efficacy, combined with a good side effect profile, translates into a better quality of life for patients given ondansetron compared with other anti-emetics [9]. Furthermore, the availability of an oral formulation of ondansetron facilitates the management of emesis in outpatients. This review summarises the clinical experience with ondansetron in the control of emesis, and its impact on quality of life in patients with breast cancer. The studies reviewed have previously been published in part or in full [5, 10–12].

Patients and Methods

Five randomised, double-blind, comparative, multicentre studies have been carried out with ondansetron in chemotherapy-naive breast cancer patients receiving cyclophosphamide-based chemotherapy regimens on an outpatient basis. These studies compared ondansetron (given as ondansetron hydrochloride dihydrate) with placebo (study 1), metoclopramide (studies 2–4) and alizapride (study 5). The number of vomits and retches, together with an assessment of nausea as none, mild, moderate or severe were recorded daily by the patients on diary cards. An emetic episode was defined as 1 vomit or 1 retch. Emesis was considered to be successfully treated in patients who experienced 2 or fewer emetic episodes (complete or major control of emesis). Nausea was successfully treated in those who graded it as none or mild (i.e. did not interfere with normal daily life).

The design of these studies and the anti-emetic dose schedules used are shown in table 1. Quality of life was formally assessed in 2 of the studies (studies 4 and 5). In study 4, quality of life was assessed using the Rotterdam Symptom Checklist (RSCL [13]). This is a ques-

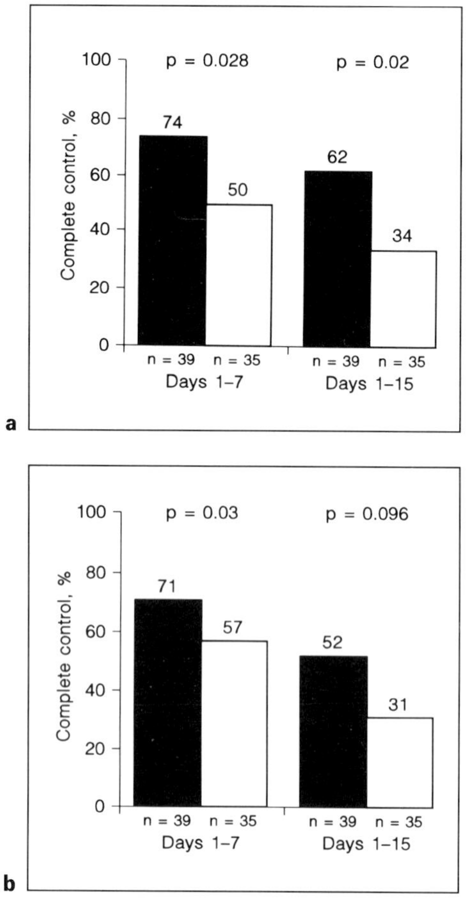

Fig. 1. Ondansetron (■) vs. placebo (□) in the control of CMF-induced emesis (**a**) and nausea (**b**).

tionnaire derived from existing questionnaires together with checklists from interviews with cancer patients. There are 38 items covering psychological and physical well-being as well as functional activity. The RSCL takes approximately 5–10 min to complete and has been validated against independent interviews. In this study, analyses were performed for the psychological, physical and functional activity subscales. Psychological (e.g. depressed) and physical (e.g. lack of energy) subscale items were graded on a scale of 0 ('not at all') to 3 ('very much'). Functional activity subscale items (e.g. care for myself) were graded in a similar manner on a scale of 0 ('unable') to 3 ('without help'). In study 5, quality of life was assessed using a general questionnaire for emesis: Functional Living Index – Cancer (FLIC [14]) and a specifically designed questionnaire for emesis: Functional Living Index – Emesis (FLIE). These questionnaires were completed before and 3 days after chemotherapy. The FLIC is a multidimensional (physical well-being and ability, emotional state, social interactions, family situation and nausea) quality of life instrument. The FLIE was modelled after the FLIC but specifically designed to assess the impact of nausea and vomiting on multiple dimensions of the patients' life.

Results

Ondansetron in the Control of CMF-Induced Emesis (Study 1)

A total of 74 patients were evaluable for efficacy: 39 of these received ondansetron and 35 were given placebo. Ondansetron was significantly superior to placebo in the complete control of emesis (0 emetic episodes) over days 1–7 and 1–15. Ondansetron prevented all emesis in 74% of patients over days 1–7 and in 62% of patients over days 1–15 while 50 and 34% of patients who received placebo did not experience emesis over days 1–7 and 1–15, respectively ($p < 0.05$; fig. 1a). Ondansetron was also superior to placebo in the control of CMF-induced nausea (fig. 1b).

Ondansetron in the Control of Acute Emesis and Nausea (Studies 2–5)

A total of 615 patients were evaluated for efficacy in these studies: 208 received ondansetron and 224 were given metoclopramide or alizapride (fig. 2–4). A further 93 and 90 patients received ondansetron plus dexamethasone and metoclopramide plus dexamethasone, respectively. Ondansetron was superior to metoclopramide or alizapride in the control of emesis and nausea over the first 24 h following FAC/FEC/EC chemotherapy (fig. 2–4). This reached statistical significance in 2 of the studies (studies 2 and 5; $p < 0.001$). Ondansetron produced a complete or major response (0–2 emetic episodes) in 72–86% of patients while metoclopramide or alizapride achieved complete or major control of emesis in 42–61% of patients (fig. 2, 4). Ondansetron when given in combination with dexamethasone was also significantly superior to metoclopramide plus dexamethasone (study 4). In this study, 96% of patients experienced 2 or fewer emetic episodes with the ondansetron regimen compared with 76% given metoclopramide plus dexamethasone (fig. 2, 3; $p < 0.001$).

Ondansetron in the Control of Delayed Emesis (Studies 2, 3 and 5)

Oral ondansetron was also superior to metoclopramide or alizapride over days 2–3/4. This reached statistical significance in 2 of the studies (studies 2 and 5; $p < 0.05$). On the 'worst day' of emesis 79–81% of ondansetron-treated patients experienced 2 or fewer emetic episodes compared with 63–65% of patients given the comparator (fig. 5).

Ondansetron in the Control of Emesis and Nausea over Repeated Courses (Study 4)

Study 4 assessed the anti-emetic response of ondansetron and metoclopramide (each with a pre-chemotherapy dose of dexamethasone) over 6 courses of chemotherapy.

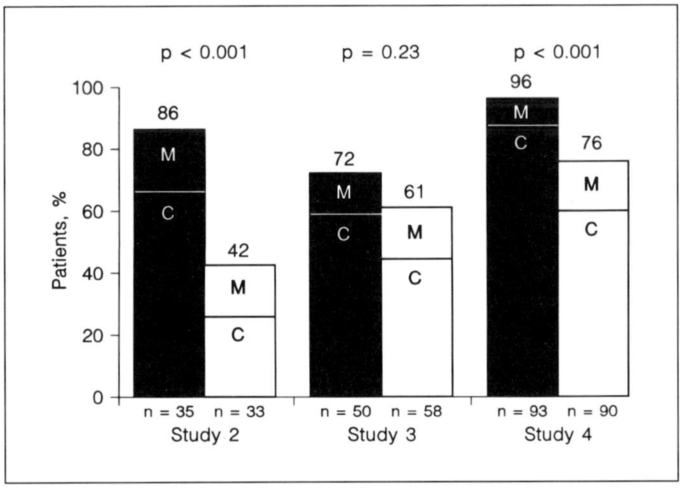

Fig. 2. Ondansetron (■) vs. metoclopramide (□) in the control of acute emesis (with a pre-chemotherapy dose of dexamethasone in study 4). C = Complete response; M = major response.

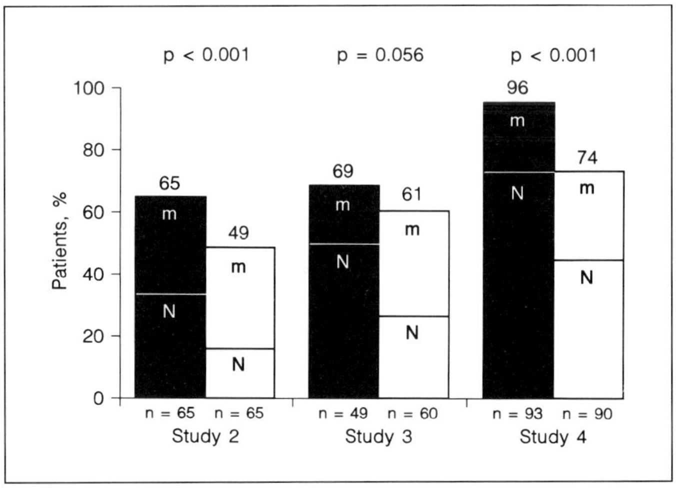

Fig. 3. Ondansetron (■) vs. metoclopramide (□) in the control of acute nausea (with a pre-chemotherapy dose of dexamethasone in study 4). N = No nausea; m = mild nausea.

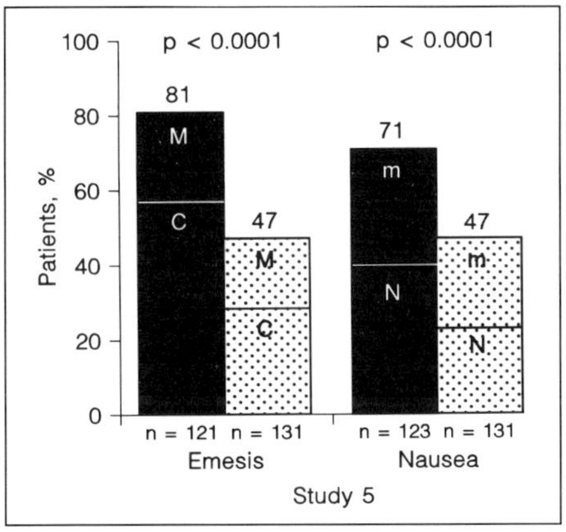

Fig. 4. Ondansetron (■) vs. alizapride (░) in the control of acute emesis and nausea. C/N = Complete response/no nausea; M/m = major response/mild nausea.

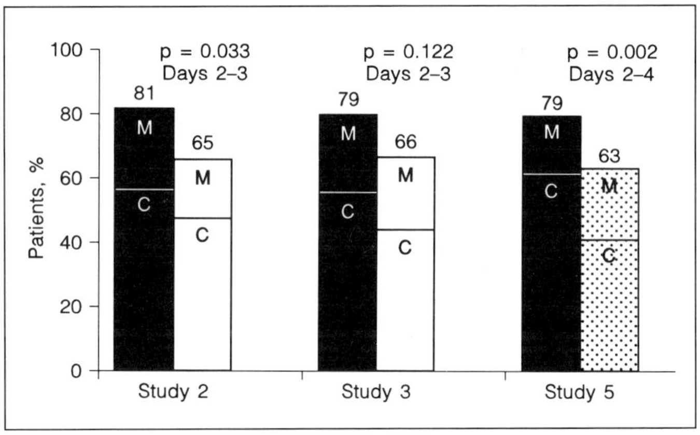

Fig. 5. Ondansetron (■) vs. metoclopramide (□) and alizapride (░) in the control of delayed emesis (worst day analysis). C = Complete response; M = major response.

Control of emesis was better maintained with ondansetron than metoclopramide (both with a pre-chemotherapy dose of dexamethasone), 67% of patients experienced 2 or fewer emetic episodes on all evaluable courses with ondansetron compared with 28% of patients given metoclopramide ($p < 0.001$; fig. 6).

Ondansetron and Quality of Life (Studies 2, 4 and 5)

Patient preference data is an important comparative parameter in studies of anti-emetics as it reflects patients' well being. Study 2 used a cross-over design allowing patients to be asked their anti-emetic preference. Significantly more patients preferred ondansetron to metoclopramide (63 vs. 26%; $p < 0.001$), although 11% of patients did not express a preference. In study 4 quality of life was assessed using the RSCL. For the first course of chemotherapy, despite starting from a higher baseline score (poorer quality of life), ondansetron significantly improved the psychological subscale scores compared with metoclopramide ($p = 0.002$). No differences were observed in the physical and functional activity subscales after the first course. Over all 6 courses of chemotherapy,

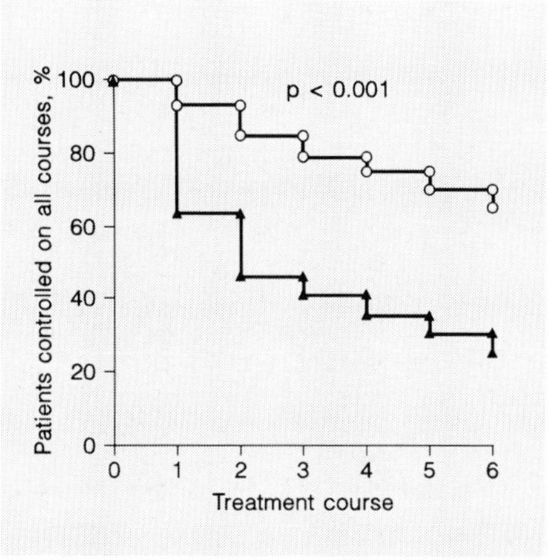

Fig. 6. Efficacy of ondansetron (○) vs. metoclopramide (▲) in the control of emesis over repeated courses (0–2 emetic episodes).

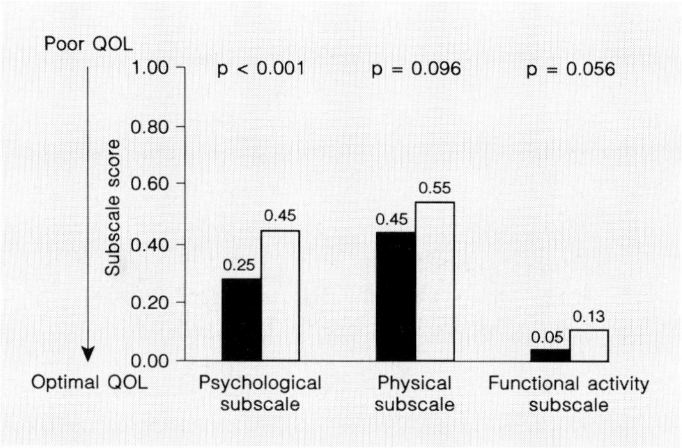

Fig. 7. Quality of life (QOL) assessments in ondansetron and metoclopramide-treated patients over 6 courses of chemotherapy using the RSCL (each with a single pre-treatment dose of dexamethasone). ■ = Ondansetron group (475 assessments); □ = metoclopramide group (380 assessments). Median post treatment subscale scores.

there was a benefit for ondansetron compared with metoclopramide on all 3 subscales which reached statistical significance for the psychological subscale (fig. 7). In study 5 there was no difference in quality of life scores between the ondansetron and alizapride groups when quality of life was measured by the FLIC; but when quality of life was measured by the FLIE, ondansetron was superior to alizapride in preventing a decrease in quality of life following chemotherapy (p = 0.04).

Adverse Events

Ondansetron was well tolerated in all of these studies. Unlike metoclopramide, ondansetron did not induce any extrapyramidal reactions. The only side effects that occurred more frequently following ondansetron administration were headache and constipation in approximately 10 and 5% of patients, respectively.

Discussion

Nausea and vomiting associated with cyclophosphamide can be severe, particularly in women [15]. The studies reviewed here have clearly shown that ondansetron is effective in the prevention of emesis and nausea following cyclophosphamide-based chemotherapy given for the treatment of breast cancer. Ondansetron is superior to placebo in the control of emesis and nausea induced by a 14-day CMF schedule. Interestingly, although CMF chemotherapy is generally regarded to be only weakly emetogenic, 50% of patients given placebo experienced emesis compared with only 26% given ondansetron.

Ondansetron was also found to be significantly superior to conventional anti-emetics (metoclopramide and alizapride) in the control of acute and delayed emesis. For acute emesis, ondansetron produced a complete or major response in 72–86% of patients compared with 42–61% given comparator anti-emetics. One of the studies combined ondansetron with a pre-chemotherapy dose of dexamethasone. Although this combination was not compared with ondansetron alone, 96% of patients given ondansetron plus dexamethasone experienced 2 or fewer emetic episodes over the first 24 h. This suggests that, as for cisplatin-induced emesis, the addition of dexamethasone enhances the efficacy of ondansetron. For delayed emesis, ondansetron was also superior to metoclopramide or alizapride. This demonstrates that oral ondansetron is effective in controlling symptoms, which is especially important in this group of patients who often receive chemotherapy on an outpatient basis. Furthermore, it is important that anti-emetic control is maintained over scheduled courses of chemotherapy which apart from helping to maintain patients' quality of life would be expected to reduce the incidence of anticipatory nausea and vomiting. One of the studies which prospectively assessed the efficacy of ondansetron over 6 courses of chemotherapy demonstrated that efficacy is well maintained and significantly superior to metoclopramide. Ondansetron was also well tolerated and unlike conventional anti-emetics, such as metoclopramide, did not induce distressing extrapyramidal reactions. These benefits of ondansetron were reflected in patient preference data and formal quality of life assessments using different questionnaires (RSCL, FLIE). In one of the studies a cross-over design was used and significantly more patients stated a preference for ondansetron over metoclopramide. Quality of life assessments used in two of the studies also showed that ondansetron is associated with a better quality of life compared with conventional anti-emetics. This has important consequences for the patient and the patient's family and may facilitate the completion of scheduled courses of chemotherapy.

Conclusions

In outpatient chemotherapy for breast cancer, ondansetron is significantly superior to both metoclopramide and alizapride in the control of acute and delayed nausea and vomiting and is better tolerated. In addition, the anti-emetic response with ondansetron is maintained over repeated courses of chemotherapy. These benefits result in a better quality of life for patients given ondansetron compared with conventional anti-emetics. The majority of breast cancer patients receive chemotherapy on an outpatient basis; the availability of an oral formulation of an effective and well tolerated anti-emetic such as ondansetron is therefore suitable for controlling nausea and vomiting in these patients.

References

1 Canellos GP, De Vita VT, Gold GL, Chabner BA, Schein PS, Young RC: Combination chemotherapy for advanced breast cancer: Response and effect on survival. Ann Intern Med 1976;84:389–392.

2 Hortobagyi GN, Body GP, Buzdar AU, Frye D, Legha SS, Malik R, Smith TL, Blumenschein GR, Yap HY, Rodriguez V: Evaluation of high-dose versus standard FAC chemotherapy for advanced breast cancer in protected environment units: A prospective randomized study. J Clin Oncol 1987;5:354–364.

3 Keiling R, Armand JP, Hurteloup P, Cappelaere P: French FAC vs FEC study in advanced breast cancer. Onkologie 1986;9(suppl 1):8–10.

4 Morran C, Smith DC, Anderson DA, McArdle CS: Incidence of nausea and vomiting with cytotoxic chemotherapy: A prospective randomized trial of antiemetics. Br Med J 1979;1:1323–1324.

5 Bonneterre J, Chevallier B, Metz R, Fargeot P, Pujade-Lauraine E, Spielmann M, Tubiana-Hulin M, Paes D, Bons J: A randomised double-blind comparison of ondansetron and metoclopramide in the prophylaxis of emesis induced by cyclophosphamide, fluorouracil and doxorubicin or epirubicin chemotherapy. J Clin Oncol 1990;8:1063–1069.

6 Marty M, Pouillart P, Scholl S, Droz JP, Azab M, Brion N, Pujade-Lauraine E, Paule B, Paes D, Bons J: Comparison of 5-hydroxytryptamine 3 (serotonin) antagonist ondansetron (GR38032F) with high-dose metoclopramide in the control of acute cisplatin-induced emesis. N Engl J Med 1990;322:816–821.

7 Roila F, Tonato M, Cognetti F, Cortesi E, Favalli G, Marangolo M, Amadori D, Bella MA, Gramazio V, Donati D, Ballatori E, Del Favero A: Prevention of cisplatin-induced emesis: A double-blind multicenter randomized crossover study comparing ondansetron and ondansetron plus dexamethasone. J Clin Oncol 1991; 9:675–678.

8 Smyth JF, Coleman RE, Nicolson M, Gallmeier WM, Leonard RCF, Cornbleet MA, Allan SG, Upadhyaya BK, Bruntsch U: Does dexamethasone enhance control of acute cisplatin-induced emesis by ondansetron? Br Med J 1991;303:1423–1426.

9 Hirsch JD, Lee JT, Grapski R: Quality of life with intravenous ondansetron vs standard anti-emetic therapy in patients receiving emetogenic cancer chemotherapy (abstract). Proc Am Soc Clin Oncol 1992;11:1368.

10 Buser K, Joss R, Piquet D, Aapro M, Cavalli F, Haefliger JM, Jungi W, Bauer J, Weber T, Verity L, Butcher M: A randomised, double-blind, placebo-controlled study of oral ondansetron in the prophylaxis of nausea and vomiting induced by chemotherapy with cyclophosphamide, methotrexate and 5-fluorouracil (CMF) in women with breast cancer (abstract). Proc Am Soc Clin Oncol 1990;9:1279.

11 Marschner NW, Adler M, Nagel GA, Christmann D, Fenzl E, Upadhyaya B: Double-blind randomized trial of the anti-emetic efficacy and safety of ondansetron and metoclopramide in advanced breast cancer patients treated with epirubicin and cyclophosphamide. Eur J Cancer 1991;27:1137–1140.

12 Soukop M, McQuade B, Hunter E, Stewart A, Kaye S, Cassidy J, Kerr D, Khanna S, Smyth J, Coleman R, Cunningham D, Powles T, Davidson N, Hutcheon A, Green J, Slater A, Rustin G, Carney D: Ondansetron compared with metoclopramide in the control of emesis and quality of life during repeated chemotherapy for breast cancer. Oncology 1992;49:295–304.

13 De Haes JCJM, Van Knippenberg FCE, Neijt JP: Measuring psychological and physical distress in cancer patients: Structure and application of the Rotterdam Symptom Checklist. Br J Cancer 1990;62:1034–1038.

14 Schipper H, Clinch J, McMurray A, Levitt M: Measuring the quality of life of cancer patients: The Functional Living Index Cancer: Development and validation. J Clin Oncol 1984;2:472–483.

15 Tonato M, Roila F, Del Favero A: Methodology of anti-emetic trials: A review. Ann Oncol 1991;2:107–114.

Oncology 1993;50:186–190

F. Cox
J. Hirsch

Glaxo Inc., Research Triangle Park, N.C., USA

Ondansetron: A Cost-Effective Advance in Anti-Emetic Therapy

Key Words
Ondansetron
Metoclopramide
Cisplatin
Cyclophosphamide
Cost-effectiveness

Abstract
A cost-effectiveness analysis is one form of full economic evaluation where drug acquisition costs and the costs that are incurred as a result of using a particular treatment are assessed together with clinical efficacy. This paper reviews two such studies. One of the studies was a prospective randomised cost-effectiveness study which compared ondansetron (8 mg i.v. 0, 4 and 8 h following chemotherapy) with metoclopramide (3 mg/kg i.v. followed by an infusion of 0.5 mg/kg/h for 8 h) over the first 24 h following chemotherapy in hospitalised patients receiving highly emetogenic chemotherapy. This study showed that the cost per successfully treated patient (defined in this study as having $\leq$ 1 emetic episode and no adverse events) for these 2 treatments were approximately equal: ondansetron £ 95 and metoclopramide £ 92. The second study was an economic evaluation based on data collected over a 5-day period following cyclophosphamide-based chemotherapy given on an outpatient basis for the treatment of breast cancer. Patients received an intravenous dose of 16 mg dexamethasone with either 8 mg ondansetron or 60 mg metoclopramide intravenously before chemotherapy followed by oral dosing with 8 mg ondansetron or 20 mg metoclopramide 3 times daily for 5 days. The costs per successfully treated patient (defined in this study as no vomiting or retching episodes and no anti-emetic-related adverse events during the 5-day period) were comparable: ondansetron £ 184 and metoclopramide £ 160. A recent study has established that ondansetron (8 mg) given orally twice daily is as effective as the same dose given 3 times a day. A sensitivity analysis using the cost of an ondansetron twice daily regimen showed that ondansetron is more cost-effective than metoclopramide (£ 133 vs. £ 160). These cost effectiveness studies have shown that ondansetron is at least as cost-effective as metoclopramide and simplified ondansetron dosing schedules render ondansetron more cost-effective. These full economic evaluations illustrate that drug acquisition costs can be a misleading guide to the economic impact of anti-emetics.

Dr. F. Cox
Glaxo Inc.
Research Triangle Park, NC 27709 (USA)

Introduction

Ondansetron is an effective and well-tolerated anti-emetic for the prevention of chemotherapy- and radiotherapy-induced nausea and vomiting [1]. However, healthcare expenditure is increasingly being subject to scrutiny and some constraint and therefore new drugs such as ondansetron must be justified not only clinically but also economically. Providers of healthcare therefore require full economic evaluations on which to base their decisions. A cost-effectiveness analysis is one form of full economic evaluation where both the cost and consequences of a healthcare programme or a treatment are examined, i.e. the acquisition costs as well as the costs that are incurred as a result of using a particular treatment are assessed together with its effectiveness [2, 3]. This paper reviews two cost-effectiveness studies that have been undertaken with ondansetron.

Study 1: Cost-Effectiveness of Ondansetron and Metoclopramide for Highly Emetogenic Chemotherapy

This prospective, randomised, cost-effectiveness study compared ondansetron and metoclopramide in hospitalised patients receiving highly emetogenic chemotherapy including cisplatin. This study has been published in full [4] and is summarised here.

Patients and Methods

This was an open, randomised parallel group pilot study. Ondansetron (as ondansetron hydrochloride dihydrate) was given as three, 8 mg intravenous doses (0, 4 and 8 h following chemotherapy). Metoclopramide was administered as a 3 mg/kg intravenous loading dose followed by an infusion of 0.5 mg/kg/h for 8 h. The number of emetic episodes and adverse events were recorded during the first 24 h. Details of all the materials used in the administration of the anti-emetics were recorded. These included 'rescue' medication needed by patients not controlled with the study drugs, medication used to treat adverse events and the time spent caring for patients who experienced emesis and adverse events. These costs were assessed together with the acquisition costs for the anti-emetics to give a utilisation cost for ondansetron and metoclopramide. Patients were considered successfully treated if they experienced no significant emesis ≤1 emetic episode) and no adverse events (fig. 1, pathway 1). The cost per successfully treated patient was obtained by dividing the mean overall cost per patient (the utilisation cost) by the probability of being successfully treated.

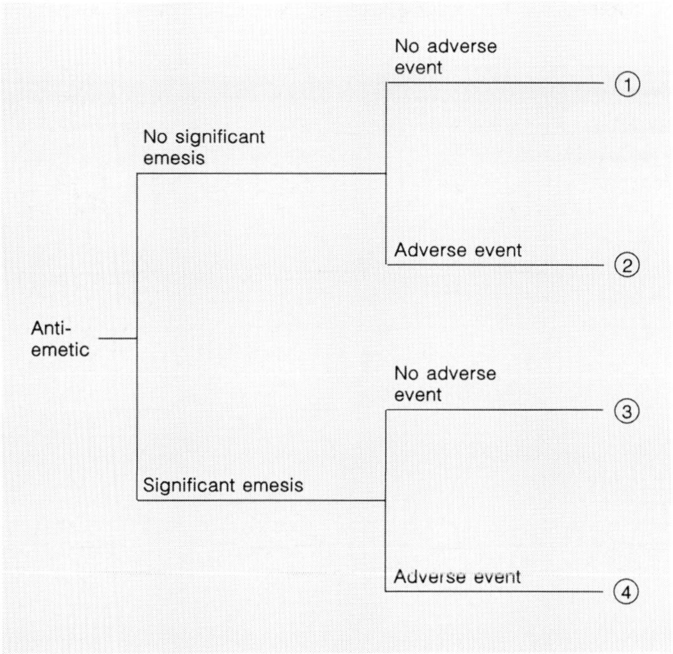

Fig. 1. Possible outcomes from anti-emetic treatment (study 1).

Table 1. Mean drug utilisation costs (in £) in the first 24 h following highly emetogenic chemotherapy

Resource item	Ondansetron n = 14	Metoclopramide n = 18
Anti-emetic drugs	44.57	11.91
Anti-emetic administration	0.26	3.74
Materials	0.73	0.59
Additional drugs	0.19	0.46
Additional drug administration	0.01	0.06
Nursing staff	1.84	3.34
Medical staff	0.00	0.18
Total	47.60	20.28

Results

Fourteen patients received ondansetron and 18 received metoclopramide. Seven of the 14 (50%) ondansetron patients were successfully treated (experienced ≤ 1 emetic episode and no adverse events) compared with 4 of the 18 (22%) patients given metoclopramide. The mean utilisation cost for ondansetron was £47.60 compared to £20.28 for metoclopramide (table 1). The costs

Table 2. Cost-effectiveness of ondansetron and metoclopramide

	Ondansetron	Metoclopramide
Number of patients	14	18
Percentage of patients successfully treated	50	22
Cost per patient, £	47.60	20.28
Cost per successfully treated patient, £	95.20	92.18

Table 3. Mean cost consequences (in £) associated with the study drugs over the 5 day period following cyclophosphamide treatment

Item	Cost
Vomiting or retching	51.24
Responding to an adverse event	20.00
Treating adverse event	5.00
Treating adverse event including hospitalisation	250.00[1]

[1] Estimated costs based on adverse event report of patient experiencing severe dystonic reaction, assumed to require only 1 night stay in hospital.

per successfully treated patient were £95.20 and £92.18 for the ondansetron and metoclopramide groups, respectively (table 2).

Study 2: Cost-Effectiveness of Ondansetron and Metoclopramide for Cyclophosphamide-Based Chemotherapy Given for the Treatment of Breast Cancer

This was a retrospective economic evaluation based on data collected over a 5-day period following chemotherapy. This evaluation used clinical trial data from a randomised, double-blind study which compared the efficacy, safety profile and impact on patients' quality of life of ondansetron and metoclopramide (each with a pre-chemotherapy dose of dexamethasone) in patients receiving cyclophosphamide-based chemotherapy on an outpatient basis for the treatment of breast cancer. The efficacy and quality of life results have previously been published [5].

Table 4. Cost per successfully treated patient for ondansetron (three times a day) and metoclopramide

Parameter	Metoclopramide	Ondansetron
Number of patients	70	80
Percentage of successfully treated patients	30	76.3
Average cost per patient, £	48.08	140.68
Cost per successfully treated patient, £	160.28	184.37

Patients and Methods

Patients received intravenous doses of dexamethasone (16 mg) with either ondansetron (8 mg i.v.) (as ondansetron hydrochloride dihydrate) or metoclopramide (60 mg i.v.) before chemotherapy, followed by oral dosing with 8 mg ondansetron (as ondansetron hydrochloride dihydrate) or 20 mg metoclopramide three times daily for 5 days following chemotherapy. Patients were not included in the analysis if they had received less than the prescribed anti-emetic regimen or low cyclophosphamide dosing. The cost-effectiveness analysis was conducted from a societal perspective using the decision tree outlined in figure 2. The average European drug costs at the time of the analysis were used and the costs associated with the consequences of drug treatment were based on actual or estimated costs derived from this study or studies with comparable patient/treatment populations [6] (table 3). These costs were then used to calculate the overall cost associated with each anti-emetic (utilisation cost).

Patients were classified as being successfully treated if they experienced no vomiting or retching episodes and no anti-emetic related adverse events during the 5-day study period (fig. 2, pathway 1). The cost-effective ratios for ondansetron and metoclopramide were then calculated by combining the costs associated with each anti-emetic and their relative efficacy.

Results

All evaluable patients (80 ondansetron and 70 metoclopramide) were included in the analysis. Seventy-six percent of patients given ondansetron were successfully treated over the 5-day study period (no vomiting or retching episodes and no anti-emetic-related adverse events) compared with 30% of patients given metoclopramide. The mean utilisation cost for ondansetron was £140.68 compared to £48.08 for metoclopramide. However, the cost per successfully treated patient for ondansetron (£184.37) was comparable to that for metoclopramide (£160.28) (table 4) despite the drug aquisition cost of ondansetron being 15 times that of metoclopramide.

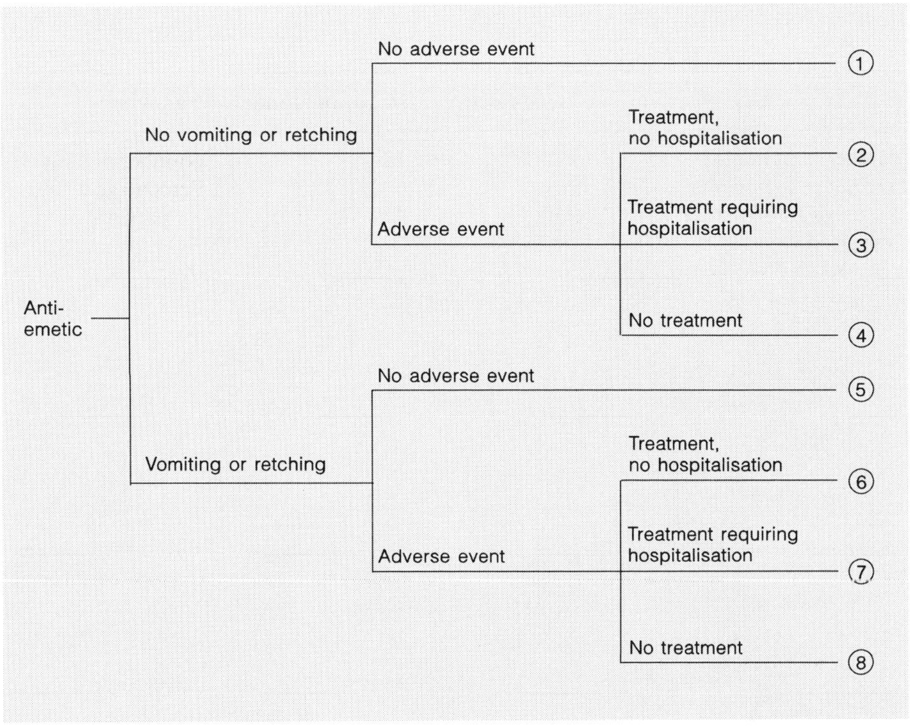

Fig. 2. Possible outcomes from anti-emetic treatment (study 2). Adverse event was defined as an event reported by the investigator as probably or almost certainly attributed to the study drug. Vomiting or retching was defined as one or more vomiting and/or retching episodes during the 5-day study period.

Sensitivity Analysis

In a separate clinical trial, it was shown that 8 mg ondansetron given orally twice daily is as effective as the same dose given three times daily in patients receiving cyclophosphamide chemotherapy [7]. The results of a sensitivity analysis which applied the costs of twice daily ondansetron dosing to the original decision tree model produced a cost per successfully treated patient for ondansetron of £133, which is less than that for metoclopramide (£160). Additional sensitivity analyses were conducted varying assumptions by as much as 20% individually and simultaneously, and the conclusions for both the three times- and twice-daily dosing models did not change.

Discussion

The two economic evaluations described here have shown that ondansetron is at least comparably cost-effective as metoclopramide. This has been demonstrated over the first 24 h following highly emetogenic chemotherapy in hospitalised patients (study 1) and over 5 days in patients receiving cyclophosphamide-based chemotherapy as outpatients for the treatment of breast cancer (study 2). These evaluations emphasise that a comparison of only drug acquisition costs can be a misleading guide to the economic impact of anti-emetic drugs. Indeed, these results indicate that the differential in acquisition price between ondansetron and metoclopramide is compensated for by the superior efficacy, lower incidence of adverse events and lower management and material costs associated with ondansetron.

The studies described here used a three-times-a-day ondansetron regimen. It is now well established that a single intravenous dose of ondansetron is effective in the control of acute emesis [8] and that an 8 mg twice daily oral regimen is as effective as the same dose given three times a day [7]. The lower drug acquisition costs of these simplified regimens may further highlight the cost-effectiveness of ondansetron relative to metoclopramide. In addition, ondansetron may also reduce the extent of emesis (i.e. the number of emetic episodes) if emesis occurs. Furthermore, ondansetron may offer significant benefits to patients as a result of avoiding emesis which is ranked by patients as the worst aspect of cancer treatment [9]. Indeed, it has been reported that patients given ondansetron have a better quality of life compared with those given metoclopramide [5].

Conclusions

In these studies ondansetron is at least as cost-effective as metoclopramide and simplified ondansetron dosing schedules may render ondansetron more cost-effective than metoclopramide. These full economic evaluations illustrate that considering only drug acquisition costs can lead to misleading and inappropriate conclusions. These studies therefore provide comprehensive information for health-care provider decision making.

References

1 Freeman AJ, Cullen MH: Advances in the management of cytotoxic drug-induced nausea and vomiting. J Clin Pharm Ther 1991;16: 411–420.

2 Bootman JL, Townsend RJ, McGhan WF: Principles of Pharmacoeconomics. Cincinnati, Harvey Whitney Books Inc, 1991.

3 Drummond MF, Stoddart GL, Torrance GW: Methods for the Economic Evaluation of Health Programme. Oxford, Oxford University Press, 1987.

4 Cunningham D, Gore M, Davidson N, Miocevich M, Manchanda M, Wells N: The real costs of emesis – An economic analysis of ondansetron vs. metoclopramide in controlling emesis in patients receiving chemotherapy for cancer. Eur J Cancer 1993;29A:303–306.

5 Soukop M, McQuade B, Hunter E, Stewart A, Kaye S, Cassidy J, Kerr D, Khanna S, Smyth J, Coleman R, Cunningham D, Powles T, Davidson N, Hutcheon A, Green J, Slater A, Rustin G, Carney D: Ondansetron compared with metoclopramide in the control of emesis and quality of life during repeated chemotherapy for breast cancer. Oncology 1992;49:295–304.

6 Buxton MJ, O'Brien BJ: Economic evaluation of ondansetron: Preliminary analysis using clinical trial data prior to price setting. Br J Cancer 1992;66(suppl XIX):S64–S67.

7 Dicato MA, Kaasa S, Campora E, Bleiberg H, Warnier P, Vindovoghel A, Cunningham D, Liebhard A, Upadhaya BK: Efficacy of twice daily versus three times daily oral ondansetron in the prevention of chemotherapy induced emesis: A randomized, single-blind, multicentre study. Clin Oncol 1992;4:275–279.

8 Brown GW, Paes D, Bryson J, Freeman AJ: The effectiveness of a single intravenous dose of ondansetron. Oncology 1992;49:273–278

9 Coates A, Abraham S, Kay SB, Sowerbutts T, Frewin C, Fox RM, Tattersall MHN: On the receiving end – Patient perception of the side effects of cancer chemotherapy. Eur J Cancer Clin Oncol 1983;19:203–208.

Oncology 1993;50:191–197

M. E. Butcher

Glaxo Group Research, Greenford, Middlesex, UK

Global Experience with Ondansetron and Future Potential

Key Words
Ondansetron
Chemotherapy-induced emesis
Delayed emesis
Dexamethasone patient
Safety profile

Abstract
Ondansetron was first synthesised in 1983 and it is estimated that over 4 million patient treatments have been given with ondansetron in clinical practice. Clinical trials in over 15,000 patients have demonstrated that ondansetron is effective and well tolerated in a range of clinical settings, including adults and children and over repeated courses of treatment. Ondansetron is convenient to administer, being effective as a single intravenous dose for the control of acute emesis and as oral therapy on a twice-daily schedule. Recent studies have also shown it to be a cost-effective anti-emetic when the costs of treatment failure of traditional anti-emetics are taken into account. Studies have also demonstrated an improved quality of life with ondansetron compared to treatment with metoclopramide. Ondansetron has also been found to be effective in the prevention or treatment of postoperative nausea and vomiting and other studies are underway to investigate its potential use in other clinical settings. Furthermore, appropriately designed trials are ongoing to evaluate the place of ondansetron in the control of cisplatin-induced delayed emesis. In conclusion, ondansetron has been shown to be a major advance in the control of nausea and vomiting associated with chemotherapy and radiotherapy.

Introduction

Ondansetron was first synthesised in 1983 and the first human subject was treated in phase I studies in 1984. The first patient was treated in 1986 with the first regulatory approval in 1990. Ondansetron hydrochloride dihydrate has now been approved for marketing in over 70 countries worldwide. A database of more than 15,000 patients treated in clinical trials currently exists, and it is estimated that in routine clinical practice more than 4 million patient treatments have been given with ondansetron. When setting out to develop a new anti-emetic for cancer patients the goal is to produce an agent with the following characteristics: (1) complete control of emesis in all treatment settings; (2) ease and convenience of use; (3) well tolerated; (4) cost-effective.

Dr. M. Butcher
Glaxo Group Research
Greenford
Middlesex UB6 OHE (UK)

Table 1. Assessment criteria

Emesis		Nausea	
Complete	no emetic episodes	None	
Major	1–2 emetic episodes	Mild	did not interfere with normal daily life
Minor	3–5 emetic episodes	Moderate	interfered with normal daily life
Failure	> 5 emetic episodes	Severe	bedridden due to nausea

1 emetic episode = 1 vomit or 1 retch.

The primary objective is to gain complete management of the patient's emesis in all clinical settings. Furthermore the anti-emetic should be easy to administer, not only for the oncologist and the nurse, but also for the patient. It should also be well tolerated and cost-effective. This review describes how ondansetron has met these criteria and outlines ongoing areas of research which are helping to further define its role in clinical practice.

Clinical Trial Design

In all studies with ondansetron carried out by Glaxo, internationally accepted efficacy criteria have been used [1] (table 1). The aim was to achieve complete control of emesis; however, for statistical purposes the complete (0 emetic episodes) and major (1–2 emetic episodes) responses were evaluated in many of the clinical trials. Nausea has been assessed on a 4-point scale: none, mild, moderate or severe. This scale focuses on how nausea affects patients' normal daily life.

In the design of clinical trials, many prognostic factors for emesis have to be taken into account [2, 3] (fig. 1). The most important of these is the cytotoxic drug given, chemotherapeutic agents vary in their emetogenicity with cisplatin being the most emetogenic. The dose and schedule of the cytotoxic drug are also important and this is further complicated by the fact that these drugs are often given in combinations. In addition, cytotoxic drugs induce different patterns of emesis, particularly in the acute phase. For example, following cisplatin maximum emesis occurs after 3–6 h [4], but with cyclophosphamide emesis is somewhat delayed with the peak of emesis being approximately 9–12 h following administration [5]. Other critical factors that have to be taken into account are gender: women experience more emesis than men, and age: young patients tend to experience more emesis than older patients following chemotherapy although this is reversed following radiotherapy. In addition, a history of motion sickness and anxiety also predisposes patients to emesis. On the other hand, chronic alcoholics tend to be protected from cytotoxic-induced emesis.

In most of the trials undertaken with ondansetron [6] only naive patients, patients who have not received chemotherapy previously, have been enrolled as a prior bad experience predisposes patients to emesis, particularly anticipatory emesis. In addition it is important to evaluate both the acute and delayed phases of emesis.

Control of Emesis in all Clinical Settings

Several recent studies have confirmed ondansetron as a highly effective anti-emetic in a wide variety of clinical settings. For example, Soukop et al. [7] have shown that in patients receiving 6 courses of cyclophosphamide-based chemotherapy on an outpatient basis for the treatment of breast cancer, approximately 90% of patients have excellent control of their emesis on each course with ondansetron plus dexamethasone. Furthermore, Roila et al. [8] have demonstrated that in patients receiving high doses of cisplatin, the acute phase of emesis is controlled with ondansetron plus dexamethasone in 80% of patients and control is maintained over subsequent courses. This study showed that this ondansetron regimen is significantly superior to metoclopramide, dexamethasone and diphenhydramine, a combination previously regarded as an optimal regimen for patients receiving high-dose cisplatin.

However, emesis can persist beyond the acute phase. This has been clearly demonstrated in a review by Lindley

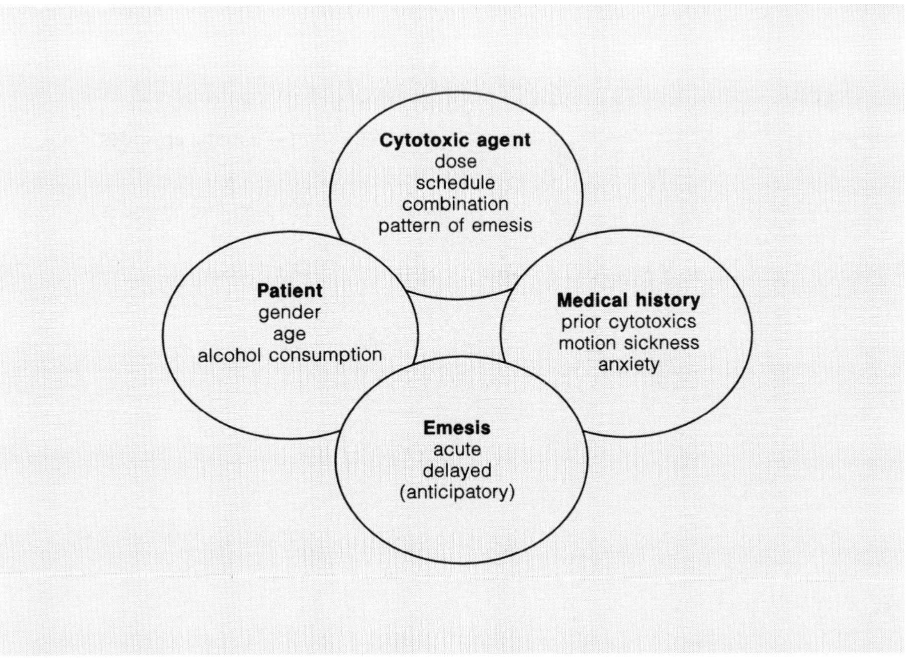

Fig. 1. Factors involved in cytotoxic-induced emesis.

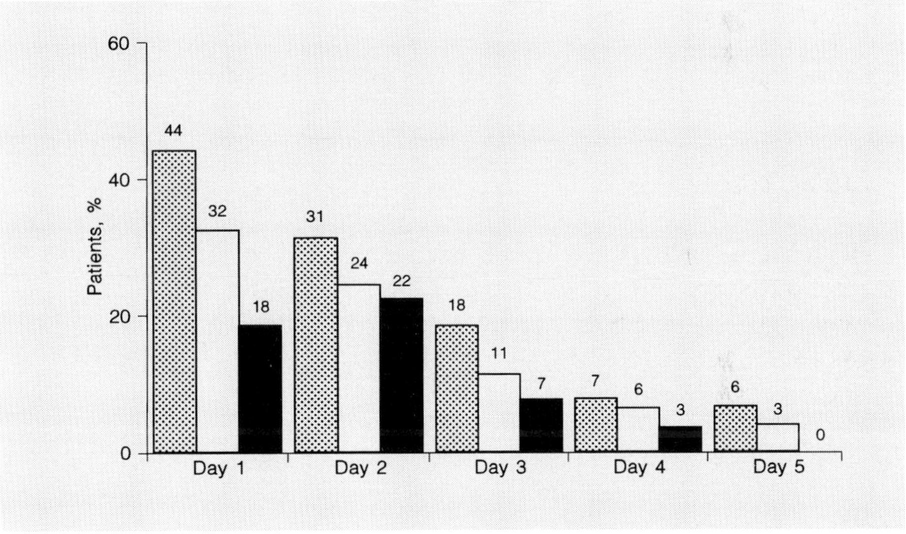

Fig. 2. The incidence of emesis despite traditional anti-emetic administration (chemotherapy on day 1 only). ▩ = Strong emetogen; □ = moderate emetogen; ■ = weak emetogen.

et al. [9], which was carried out before the 5-HT_3 receptor antagonists were available (fig. 2). In approximately 100 patients receiving 'strong', 'moderate' or 'weakly' emetogenic chemotherapy, both nausea and vomiting occurred for up to 5 days. This was despite conventional anti-emetics being taken by the majority of patients. It is important therefore that patients receive effective anti-emetic cover to control delayed emesis. Indeed, data from a meta-analysis carried out in patients receiving non-cisplatin chemotherapy has demonstrated the superiority of oral ondansetron over metoclopramide [10] (fig. 3).

Many studies have attempted to evaluate anti-emetics in the control of cisplatin-induced delayed emesis. Some clinical trial results have indicated that ondansetron and other 5-HT_3 receptor antagonists may be no more effective than conventional agents in this situation [11]. However, there are design flaws in many of these studies, for example they are often not sized appropriately and patients are not randomised at the end of the acute phase (24 h). This is important, as patients who are well controlled on the first day following chemotherapy may have less emesis on subsequent days. Futhermore, patients who

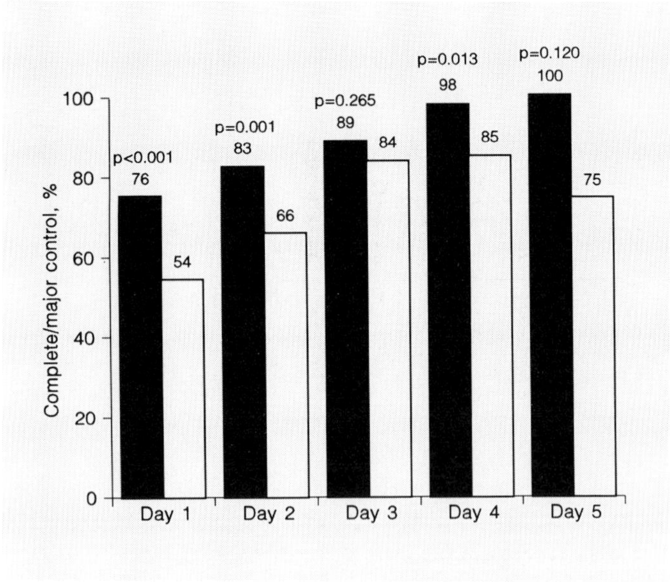

Fig. 3. Ondansetron (■) vs. metoclopramide (□) for the control of delayed emesis following non-cisplatin chemotherapy (a meta-analysis).

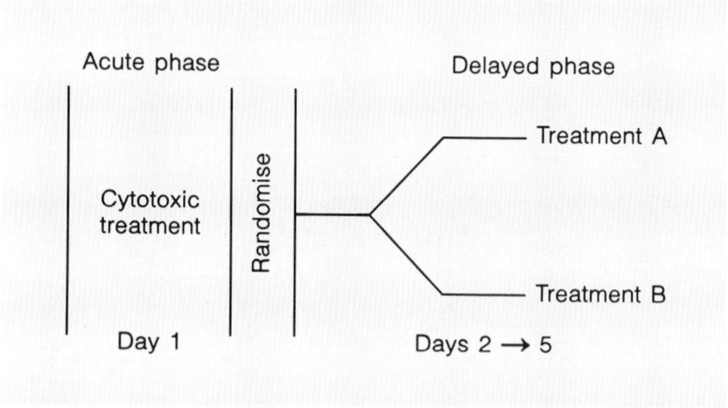

Fig. 4. Ideal study design to evaluate anti-emetics in delayed emesis.

experience severe emesis or adverse events may be withdrawn from the study on day 1, so the groups are not comparable for the delayed phase. A small study by Gandara [12], the only study where patients have been randomised after the first 24 h, compared ondansetron with placebo in patients receiving very high doses of cisplatin $\geqslant 100$ mg/m²). This study indicated that ondansetron has efficacy in the control of delayed emesis. Indeed, further large studies with ondansetron are underway utilising this study design (fig. 4).

Ease and Convenience of Use

Ondansetron is available both in intravenous and oral forms. It may therefore be taken at home as well as in the hospital, with obvious benefits enabling patients to continue with their normal daily activities and maintain their quality of life. Futhermore, ondansetron can be given as a single intravenous dose [13] before chemotherapy to control acute emesis or as a twice daily oral schedule [14].

Tolerability

Ondansetron has also been shown to be well tolerated [15]. In over 8,000 cancer patients in clinical trials approximately 11% suffered from transient headache, usually mild, and constipation has been observed in approximately 7% of patients. However, evaluating the safety profile of a new drug in cancer patients is difficult due to the high 'background noise' of adverse events due to other factors. A large clinical database now exists in non-cancer patients, primarily surgical patients receiving ondansetron for postoperative nausea and vomiting. In these patients, the adverse event profile for ondansetron is similar to placebo [16]. Of particular importance to cancer patients, ondansetron is not associated with acute dystonic reactions unlike dopamine receptor antagonists such as metoclopramide.

Cost Effectiveness

Measures of the cost-effectiveness of a new drug are becoming increasingly important [17]. Cox and Hirsch [18] have presented results from a cost-effectiveness model in breast cancer patients showing that ondansetron is similarly cost-effective to metoclopramide. This model looks beyond simple acquisition costs to evaluate the costs associated with the consequences of treatment failure and side effects. Other studies have also shown ondansetron to be a cost-effective anti-emetic in other clinical situations [19].

Future Potential

Currently three 5-HT_3 receptor antagonists, ondansetron, granisetron and tropisetron, are available in some countries. In ferrets all three agents can effectively prevent emesis, but at present there are no trials in man comparing these agents in appropriately designed clinical trials. An extensive review of the literature shows a range of efficacy for these agents although at present there is little published data for tropisetron [4, 11, 20–45] (fig. 5, 6). As efficacy will depend on the many prognostic factors for emesis, only direct head-to-head comparisons will reveal the benefits, if any, that one 5-HT_3 receptor antagonist may have over another.

The benefits of ondansetron using measures other than the control of emesis are also being evaluated. A study in breast cancer patients has shown that the use of ondansetron to prevent emesis over 6 courses of non-cisplatin chemotherapy is associated with a better quality of life for patients compared with metoclopramide [7]. This trial assessed quality of life using the Rotterdam Symptom Checklist. Further studies with ondansetron are currently underway using other quality of life instruments such as the Functional Living Index – Cancer (FLIC) and Functional Living Index – Emesis (FLIE) questionnaires, in patients receiving high doses of cisplatin.

Ondansetron has also been studied in clinical settings other than for the control of cytotoxic-induced emesis. For example, the first regulatory approvals for the use of ondansetron hydrochloride dihydrate in the prevention or treatment of postoperative nausea and vomiting have now been obtained [46].

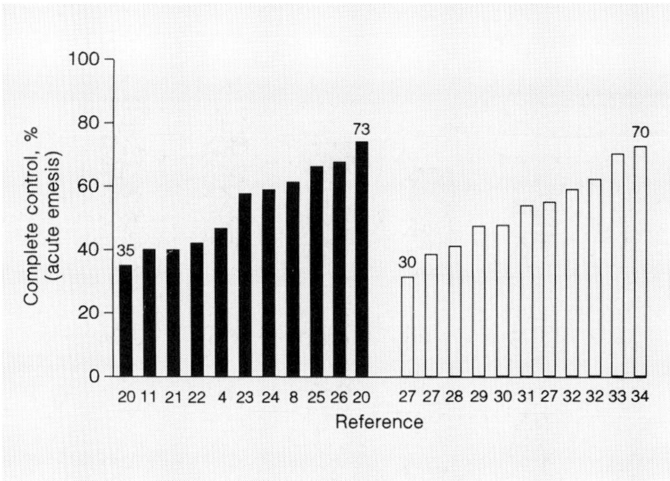

Fig. 5. Comparison of the efficacy of ondansetron (■) and granisetron (□) against highly emetogenic chemotherapy (based on published comparative trials).

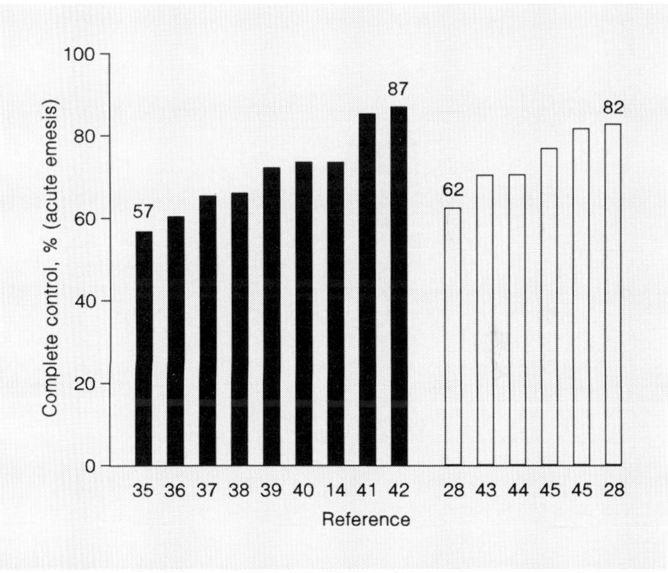

Fig. 6. Comparison of efficacy of ondansetron (■), granisetron (□) and tropisetron against non-cisplatin chemotherapy (based on published comparative trials).

Conclusions

When setting out to develop a new anti-emetic the goal was to produce an agent that completely controlled emesis in all treatment settings which was convenient to administer, well tolerated and cost-effective. This review has assessed how ondansetron has met these criteria.

Ondansetron hydrochloride dihydrate is effective in a range of treatment settings, including cisplatin, non-cisplatin and radiotherapy-induced emesis, furthermore this efficacy is maintained over repeated courses of treatment. Children are particularly susceptible to severe emesis following chemotherapy and again ondansetron is effective in this group. However, ondansetron does not completely abolish emesis in all patients although the addition of dexamethasone improves efficacy. Ondansetron is also well tolerated and convenient to administer being effective as a single intravenous dose for the control of acute emesis and as oral therapy on a twice daily schedule. Finally, two recent studies have shown that ondansetron is cost-effective for both cisplatin and non-cisplatin induced emesis.

Thus, ondansetron is a major advance in the control of emesis in cancer patients, although the truly 'ideal' anti-emetic remains an elusive goal. However, future studies will further define the role of ondansetron in clinical practice.

References

1 Gralla RJ, Itri LM, Pisko SE, Squillante AE, Kelsen DP, Braun DW, Bordin LA, Braun TJ, Young CW: Antiemetic efficacy of high-dose metoclopramide: Randomised trials with placebo and prochlorperazine in patients with chemotherapy-induced nausea and vomiting. N Engl J Med 1981;305:905–909.

2 Olver IN, Simon RN, Aisner J: Antiemetic studies: A methodological discussion. Cancer Treat Rev 1986;70:555–563.

3 Olver IN: Antiemetic study design: Desirable objectives, stratifications and analyses. Br J Cancer 1992;66(suppl 19):S30–S34.

4 Marty M, Pouillart P, Scholl S, Droz JP, Azab M, Brion N, Pujade-Lauraine E, Paule B, Paes D, Bons J: Comparison of the 5-hydroxytryptamine 3 (serotonin) antagonist ondansetron (GR 38032F) with high-dose metoclopramide in the control of cisplatin-induced emesis. N Engl J Med 1990;322:816–821.

5 Fetting JH, Grochow LB, Folstein MF: The course of nausea and vomiting after high-dose cyclophosphamide. Cancer Treat Rev 1982;66: 1487–1493.

6 Proceedings of the Ondansetron Symposium, Queen Elizabeth II Conference Centre, London, June 1989. Eur J Cancer Clin Oncol 1989; 25:(suppl 1):S3–S93.

7 Soukop M, McQuade B, Hunter E, Stewart A, Kaye S, Cassidy J, Kerr D, Khanna S, Smyth J, Coleman R, Cunningham D, Powles T, Davidson N, Hutcheon A, Green J, Slater A, Rustin G, Carney D: Ondansetron compared with metoclopramide in the control of emesis and quality of life during repeated chemotherapy for breast cancer. Oncology 1992;49:295–304.

8 Roila F, Italian Group for Antiemetic Research: Ondansetron plus dexamethasone vs metoclopramide plus dexamethasone plus diphenhydramine in the prevention of cisplatin-induced emesis. Lancet 1992;340:96–99.

9 Lindley CM, Bernard D, Fields SM: Incidence and duration of chemotherapy-induced nausea and vomiting in the outpatient oncology population. J Clin Oncol 1987;7:1142–1149.

10 Schmoll HJ: The role of ondansetron in the treatment of emesis induced by non-cisplatin-containing chemotherapy regimens. Eur J Cancer Clin Oncol 1989;25(suppl 1):S35–S39.

11 De Mulder P, Seyenaeve C, Vermorken JB, van Liessum PA, Mols-Jevdevic S, Lane Allman E, Beranek P, Verweij J: Ondansetron compared with high-dose metoclopramide in the prophylaxis of acute and delayed cisplatin-induced nausea and vomiting – A multicentre randomised, double-blind, crossover study. Ann Intern Med 1990;113:834–840.

12 Gandara D: Progress in the control of acute and delayed emesis induced by cisplatin. Eur J Cancer 1991;27(suppl 1):S9–S11.

13 Brown GW, Paes D, Bryson J, Freeman AJ: The effectiveness of a single intravenous dose of ondansetron. Oncology 1992;49:273–278.

14 Dicato MA, Kaasa S, Campora E, Bleiberg H, Warnier P, Vindovoghel A, Cunningham D, Liebhard A, Upadhyaya BK: Efficacy of twice daily versus three times daily oral ondansetron in the prevention of chemotherapy induced emesis: A randomised, single-blind, multicentre study. Clin Oncol 1992;4:275–279.

15 Smith RN: Safety of ondansetron. Eur J Cancer Clin Oncol 1989;25(suppl):S47-S50.

16 Castle WM, Jukes AJ, Griffiths CJ, Roden SM, Greenstreet YLA: Safety of ondansetron. Eur J Anaesthesiol 1992;9(suppl 6):63–66.

17 Buxton MJ, O'Brien BJ: Economic evaluation of ondansetron: Preliminary analysis using clinical trial data prior to price setting. Br J Cancer 1992;66 (suppl 19):S64–S67.

18 Cox F, Hirsch J: Ondansetron – A cost-effective advance in anti-emetic therapy. Oncology 1993;50:186–190.

19 Cunningham D, Gore M, Davidson N, Miocevich M, Manchanda M, Wells N: The real costs of emesis – An economic analysis of ondansetron vs. metoclopramide in controlling emesis in patients receiving chemotherapy for cancer. Eur J Cancer 1993;29A:303–306.

20 Beck TM, Hesketh PJ, Madajewicz S, Navari RM, Pendergrass K, Lester EP, Kish JA, Murphy WK, Hainsworth JD, Gandara DR, Bricker LJ, Keller AM, Mortimer J, Galvin DV, House KW, Bryson JC: Stratified, randomised, double-blind comparison of intravenous ondansetron administered as a multiple-dose regimen versus two single-dose regimens in the prevention of cisplatin-induced nausea and vomiting. J Clin Oncol 1992;10:1969–1975.

21 Hainsworth J, Harvey W, Pendergrass K, Kasimis B, Oblon D, Monaghan G, Gandara D, Hesketh P, Khojasteh A, Harker G, York M, Siddiqui T, Finn A: A single-blind comparison of intravenous ondansetron, a selective serotonin antagonist, with intravenous metoclopramide in the prevention of nausea and vomiting associated with high-dose cisplatin chemotherapy. J Clin Oncol 1991;9:721–728.

22 Smyth JF, Coleman RE, Nicolson M, Gallmeier WM, Leinard RCF, Cornbleet MA, Allan SG, Upadhyaya BK, Bruntsch U: Does dexamethasone enhance control of acute cisplatin induced emesis by ondansetron? Br J Med 1991;303:1423–1426.

23 Seynaeve C, Schuller J, Buser K, Porteder H, Van Belle S, Sevelda P, Christmann D, Schmidt M, Kitchener H, Paes D, de Mulder PHM: Comparison of the anti-emetic efficacy of different doses of ondansetron, given as either a continuous infusion or a single intravenous dose, in acute cisplatin-induced emesis. A multicentre, double-blind, randomised, parallel group study. Br J Cancer 1992;66:192–197.

24 Marty M, d'Allens H: Double-blind multicentre study of 2 dose schedules of intravenous ondansetron in the control of cisplatin-induced emesis: Single dose vs continuous infusion. Cah Cancer 1990;2:541–546.

25 Chevallier B, Marty M: A double blind randomised study to compare the efficacy and safety of ondansetron versus ondansetron plus methylprednisolone in combination in the prophylaxis of cisplatin induced emesis (abstract 698). Ann Oncol 1992;3:182.

26 Depierre A, Lebeau B, d'Allens H: A comparison of ondansetron with alizapride plus methylprednisolone in the control of cisplatin-induced emesis. Oncology 1992;49:305–311.

27 Schneider M: Incidence of delayed cisplatin-induced emesis following acute anti-emetic prophylaxis with granisetron: A historical review (abstract). SmithKline Beecham Satellite Symp, 15th Int Cancer Congr, Hamburg, 1990, pp 19–21.

28 Bots MWPG, Dijkstra HJ, Biljham GH, van der Wall E, Fehmers MCO, Keizer HJ, Nortier JWR, Siegenbeek van Heukelom L, Slee PH, Veenhof CHN: A randomised trial of two doses of granisetron in the treatment of chemotherapy-induced emesis. Dutch results within a multinational study. Neth J Med 1992;40:221–226.

29 Venner P: Control of cisplatin-induced nausea and vomiting: A double-blind comparative study (abstract). Smithkline Beecham Symp, 15th Int Cancer Congr, Hamburg, 1990, pp 11–13.

30 Warr D, Wilan A, Venner P, Pater J, Kaizer L, Laberge F, Latreille J, Stewart D, O'Connell G, Osoba D, Wilson K, Davis A, Johnston D: A randomised, double-blind comparison of granisetron with high-dose metoclopramide, dexamethasone and diphenhydramine for cisplatin-induced emesis. Eur J Cancer 1993;29A:33–31.

32 Bleiberg H: Control of acute emesis with granisetron (abstract). SmithKline Beecham Satellite Symp, 17th Congr Eur Soc Med Oncol, Lyon, 1992, pp 12–16.

32 Soukop M: A comparison of two dose levels of granisetron in patients receiving high-dose cisplatin. Eur J Cancer 1990;26 (suppl 1):S15–S19.

33 Kamanabrou D: Intravenous granisetron-establishing the optimal dose. Eur J Cancer 1992; 28A (suppl 1):S6–S11.

34 Chevallier B: Efficacy and safety of granisetron compared with high-dose metoclopramide in patients receiving high-dose cisplatin in a single-blind study. Eur J Cancer 1990;26(suppl 1):S33–S36.

35 Bonneterre J, Clavel M, the Ondansetron Breast Cancer Study Group: Comparison between ondansetron tablet and alizapride injection in the prevention of emesis induced by cytotoxic regimens in breast cancer patients (abstract 699). Ann Oncol 1992;3:183.

36 Marschner N: Anti-emetic control with ondansetron in the chemotherapy of breast cancer: A review. Eur J Cancer 1991;27(suppl 1):S15–S17.

37 Kaasa S, Kvaloy S, Dicato MA, Ries F, Huys JV, Royer E, Carruthers L: A comparison of ondansetron with metoclopramide in the prophylaxis of chemotherapy induced nausea and vomiting: A randomized, double-blind study. Eur J Cancer 1990;26:311–314.

38 Bonneterre J, Chevallier B, Metz R, Fargeot P, Pujade-Lauraine E, Spielmann M, Tubiana-Hulin M, Paes D, Bons J: A randomised double-blind comparison of ondansetron and metoclopramide in the prophylaxis of emesis induced by cyclophosphamide, fluorouracil and doxorubicin or epirubicin chemotherapy. J Clin Oncol 1990;8:1063–1069.

39 Harousseau JL, Gisselbrecht C, Paillarse JM: Comparison of ondansetron and alizapride in the prophylaxis of lymphoma chemotherapy-induced emesis; in Marty M, Pappo M (eds): Ondansetron and Chemotherapy Induced Emesis. 3rd Int Congr on Neo-Adjuvant Chemotherapy. Springer-Verlag, France, 1991, pp 9–22.

40 Jones AL, Cunningham D, Soukop M, Hutcheon AW, Cassidy J, Kaye SB, Sikora K, Carney DN, Cunningham D: Dexamethasone is as effective as ondansetron in the prophylaxis of emesis induced by moderately emetogenic chemotherapy. Lancet 1991;338:483–487.

41 Fraschini G, Ciociola A, Esparza L, Templeton D, Holmes FA, Walters RS, Hortobagyi GN: Evaluation of three oral doses of ondansetron in the prevention of nausea and emesis associated with cyclophosphamide-doxorubicin chemotherapy. J Clin Oncol 1991;9:1268–1274.

42 NCIC Clinical Trials Group: An assessment of the antiemetic efficacy, tolerance and safety of GR 38032F vs dexamethasone plus metoclopramide in patients with breast cancer receiving CMF chemotherapy. Proc Natl Cancer Inst Can 1991;6:333–349.

43 Marty M: A comparative study of the use of granisetron, a selective 5-HT_3 receptor antagonist, versus a standard anti-emetic regimen of chlorpromazine plus dexamethasone in the treatment of cytostatic-induced emesis. Eur J Cancer 1990;26 (suppl 1):S26–S32.

44 Warr D, Willan A, Fine S, Wilson K, Davis A, Erlichman C, Rusthoven J, Lofters W, Osoba D, Laberge F, Latreille J, Pater J: Superiority of granisetron to dexamethasone plus prochlorperazine in the prevention of chemotherapy-induced emesis. J Natl Cancer Inst 1991;83: 1169–1173.

45 Smith IE: A comparison of two dose levels of granisetron in patients receiving moderately emetogenic cytostatic chemotherapy. Eur J Cancer 1990;26(suppl 1):S19–S23.

46 Ondansetron in post-operative nausea and vomiting; in Vickers MD, Cunningham K (eds): Proc Symp held at the Queen Elizabeth II Conference Centre, London, February 1992. Eur J Anaesth 1992;9(suppl 6):1–69.

Oncology 1993;50:198–199

M. Soukop
Royal Infirmary, Glasgow, UK

Summary and Conclusions

Ondansetron Clinical Experience

Since ondansetron was launched over 3 years ago over 1 million patients have been treated. This sizeable and rapidly growing database has confirmed the effectiveness, and most importantly, the safety profile of ondansetron. Professor Marty hypothesised that this combination of efficacy and tolerability might allow us, with the use of chemoprotective agents, to increase the doses of cytotoxic drugs used and thereby enhance their therapeutic effectiveness. This is certainly a possible future development resulting from the use of these new agents.

Ondansetron Dosing Regimens

Ondansetron is effective when given as a single intravenous dose prior to chemotherapy followed by twice daily oral dosing. It is therefore easy and convenient to use for inpatients and outpatients. Indeed, the majority of chemotherapy regimens are given on an outpatient basis.

Ondansetron plus Dexamethasone

Dr. Rath and Dr. Roila showed that the combination of ondansetron plus dexamethasone represents a very effective treatment option for cisplatin-induced emesis. This combination is significantly superior to anti-emetic combinations previously thought to be optimal: metoclopramide plus dexamethasone and metoclopramide plus dexamethasone and diphenhydramine. Indeed, the use of ondansetron plus dexamethasone should not only be considered for patients receiving cisplatin chemotherapy but also patients given agents such as cyclophosphamide which can induce severe emesis, particularly in women.

Ondansetron in Radiotherapy-Induced Emesis

Ondansetron is effective in the control of emesis induced by a variety of radiotherapy schedules. Dr. Roberts described two comparative studies in which ondansetron was shown to be superior to conventional anti-emetics in the control of emesis induced by single high-dose radiotherapy and fractionated radiotherapy. Data was also presented which showed that ondansetron is effective in patients receiving total body and hemi-body irradiation. Anecdotal data was also presented which showed that ondansetron is able to 'switch off' established emesis when used for the treatment of radiotherapy-induced emesis.

Impact of Ondansetron on Patients' Quality of Life

The quality of life of patients with cancer and undergoing chemotherapy treatment is an important consideration for the oncologist. Studies which formally assess patients' quality of life using validated instruments provide useful information which enable us to select appropriate treatment strategies. Studies using ondansetron which have assessed the quality of life of breast cancer patients have shown that ondansetron is not only associated with superior efficacy and tolerability but also with a better quality of life compared with standard anti-emetics.

Dr. M. Soukup
Royal Infirmary
Glasgow (UK)

Cost-Effectiveness of Ondansetron

Dr. Cox presented data from a prospective cost-effectiveness study which compared ondansetron with metoclopramide in hospitalised patients receiving highly emetogenic chemotherapy. Data was also presented using an economic model applied to patients receiving cyclophosphamide-based chemotherapy for the treatment of breast cancer on an outpatient basis. These evaluations showed that the cost-effectiveness ratios of ondansetron and metoclopramide in these situations are approximately equal. These studies used a three times-a-day ondansetron dosing schedule. The simplified ondansetron dosing schedules that have been established may render ondansetron more cost-effective than metoclopramide in these situations.

Global Experience and Future Directions

Dr. Butcher reviewed the ondansetron database, emphasing that ondansetron gives excellent control of nausea and emesis in a number of clinical situations in the cancer field (e.g., testicular cancer, breast cancer, paediatrics) and also emesis induced by a variety of other stimuli such as postoperative nausea and vomiting. Future studies will further define the role of ondansetron in these clinical settings.

Conclusions

The objective of this symposium was to review the large ondansetron clinical database that now exists and discuss the latest clinical trial results. These data have shown that ondansetron is a highly effective and well-tolerated anti-emetic and will help clinicians to use this agent in an optimal manner.

Special Issue
Included in subscription

Oncology (ISSN 0030–2414), **Vol. 49, No. 4 (1992)**
Editors: P.P. Carbone, Madison, Wisc.; S. Eckhardt, Budapest, K. Munk, Heidelberg, G.P. Murphy, Atlanta, Ga.; H. Sugano, Tokyo; H. Wrba, Vienna

Ondansetron –
A New Concept in Anti-Emetic Therapy

Satellite Symposium Held during the Sixth European Conference on Clinical Oncology and Cancer Nursing
Florence, October 27–31, 1991

Editors:

J. Smyth, Edinburgh

K. Cunningham, Greenford

This publication provides up-to-date information on the use of the anti-emetic ondansetron, the first 5-HT_3 receptor antagonist to be developed and marketed. Leading specialists discuss the physiology of post-chemotherapy emesis, and present the results of clinical studies regarding simplified dosing schedules of ondansetron as well as its superior efficacy compared with other anti-emetic drugs. Further papers are concerned with the methodology of clinical studies including the problem of assessing the patients' quality of life. Finally, the nurse's perspective regarding the management of emesis following chemotherapy is evaluated. In summary, this collection of data shows that ondansetron is an effective and well-tolerated anti-emetic for both adult and pediatric patients receiving emetogenic cancer treatment.

Contents

Fields of Interest
Oncology, Pharmacology

Ondansetron – A New Concept in Anti-Emetic Therapy
Satellite Symposium Held during the Sixth European Conference on Clinical Oncology and Cancer Nursing
Florence, October 27–31, 1991
'Oncology', Vol. 49, No. 4 (1992)
Editors: Smyth, J. (Edinburgh); Cunningham, K. (Greenford)
64 p., 24 fig., 10 tab., soft cover, 1992
SFr. 102.– / DM 122.– / US$ 81.75
Prices subject to change · DM price for FRG, US$ price for USA only
ISBN 3-8055-5656-X

KI 92160

KARGER